D0197792

ADVANCE PRAISE

"Diving accidents in shallow water happen. In 2011, O'Brien dove into seemingly deep water. It was a simple plummet into a wave. No swimmer could have predicted that a sand bar had moved in with the tide. It changed his life forever. A moving sand bar can shift. It was O'Brien's bad luck that it did.

"Author Meg McGovern notes that every year approximately 1,800 swimmers have diving accidents resulting in spinal cord injuries. This inspiring book should be given to people in SCI rehab centers everywhere to encourage them to gain control over their lives. O'Brien has come a long way; with determination, they can too."

MIMS CUSHING
Book reviewer, The Florida Times-Union

Stay determined!
meg mcgovern

We're Good

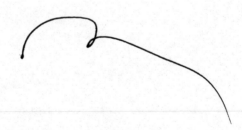

Contact me for an event/books:
mkmcgovern18@gmail.com
www.megkmcgovern.com/
Please write a review
amazon.com/author/megkeeshanmcgovern

WE'RE GOOD

The Power of Faith, Hope, and Determination

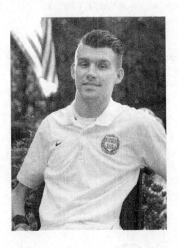

Meg Keeshan McGovern

NEW YORK

LONDON • NASHVILLE • MELBOURNE • VANCOUVER

WE'RE GOOD

The Power of Faith, Hope, and Determination

© 2019 Meg Keeshan McGovern

All rights reserved. No portion of this book may be reproduced, stored in a retrieval system, or transmitted in any form or by any means—electronic, mechanical, photocopy, recording, scanning, or other—except for brief quotations in critical reviews or articles, without the prior written permission of the publisher.

Published in New York, New York, by Morgan James Publishing. Morgan James is a trademark of Morgan James, LLC. www.MorganJamesPublishing.com

The Morgan James Speakers Group can bring authors to your live event. For more information or to book an event visit The Morgan James Speakers Group at www.TheMorganJamesSpeakersGroup.com.

Verses marked GNB are taken from Good News Bible, Today's English Version copyright © 1992, The American Bible Society, New York, NY 10023.

ISBN 9781683509134 paperback
ISBN 9781683509141 eBook
Library of Congress Control Number: 2017919153

Cover Design by:
Christopher Kirk
www.GFSstudio.com

Author and Cover Photos by:
Dana DeTullio Bauro

Interior Design by:
Chris Treccani
www.3dogcreative.net

Drawings by:
David Mitchell and Matthew O'Brien

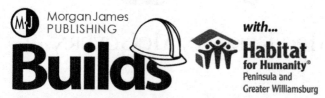

In an effort to support local communities, raise awareness and funds, Morgan James Publishing donates a percentage of all book sales for the life of each book to Habitat for Humanity Peninsula and Greater Williamsburg.

Get involved today! Visit
www.MorganJamesBuilds.com

For my father,
William F. Keeshan, Jr. (May 21, 1934 – July 15, 2016),
and my mother, Jacqueline C. Keeshan.

My father was *my* anchor.
He always believed in me and encouraged me to pursue my dreams,
one of which was to write this book.

My mother is *my* rose.
She continues to amaze me with her faith and hope despite the loss
of my dad, her husband of fifty-eight years.

ACKNOWLEDGEMENTS

Writing this book has been an amazing journey. It all began at a holiday party in 2014 when I was catching up with Carrie, a longtime friend and Chris's mom. As always, I asked how Chris was doing, which led to my question, "When is Chris going to write his story?" When Carrie responded that Chris had no plans, I said matter-of-factly, "Then I'll write it for him." And so it was that Chris, Carrie, sometimes Paul, and I began meeting weekly after work, Chris either in his chair or standing frame, Carrie often cooking dinner, and me at the counter with my computer, tape recorder, and a list of questions. Sometimes a friend or family member would stop in and offer thoughts and feelings over a glass of wine. The hours would just fly by, Chris telling me the details of his accident, about his emotions, his rehabilitation, work, studies through Harvard University's Extension School, and of course his immediate goals and those for the future. There were times when we'd be in tears together and times we'd be laughing hysterically.

Writing *We're Good* has truly been a family affair for the O'Briens and perhaps even a bit of therapy for everyone involved. From immediate family members including Chris's brother Matt, grandparents, aunts, and cousins to friends, coaches, and people he met in rehabilitation, this book is a compilation of the many lives touched and inspired by Chris's life. *We're Good* is a collective effort among those willing to share with me their relationship with Chris and how his accident impacted their own lives. Wearing their hearts on their sleeves, they opened up about their personal weaknesses and how Chris made them stronger people.

In particular, I want to thank Kiera and Alicia and their family, who shared the challenges faced when Shaun, a brother and son, became a paraplegic. They are now grieving the loss of Shaun, who passed away in October 2017. My wish is that they continue to find strength through Chris's faith, hope, and determination.

I want to thank Matthew O'Brien for his drawing ideas and David Mitchell, Chris's grandpa, for his intricate artwork that ties together symbolism in the book so beautifully, and Dana DeTullio Bauro for her professional photographs of Chris and me.

I'd be remiss not to thank my husband, Brian, and sons Billy and Peter, who encouraged and supported me to continue writing even when I became overwhelmed with other responsibilities, especially teaching. They stepped in to take care of household chores, and thankfully Brian likes to cook for all of us, otherwise dinner might not have made it to the table.

A special thanks goes to my editor, Angie Kiesling of The Editorial Attic, who spent hours reading, editing, and conferring with me to fine-tune *We're Good*. Also a huge thanks goes to Morgan James Publishing including Justin Bartlett who initially responded to my query, David Hancock the Founder of Morgan James, Jim Howard the Publisher, Gayle West my Author Relations Manager, the design team and the marketing team who have guided me through the publishing process.

Lastly, and most importantly, I want to thank Chris for having the faith in *me* to write *his* story. Even when I asked difficult and deep questions, Chris was willing to share his innermost self, which is what makes *We're Good* so powerful. In this process, I too grew stronger as a person and fulfilled my dream as a writer. The bond we have created is life changing and one I will cherish forever.

CONTENTS

MOONDANCE   xiii

Preface   Nearly Drowning   xv

PART I   **CHOOSING LIFE**   **1**

Chapter 1   God's Plan   3

Chapter 2   Chris   9

Chapter 3   Swimming at the College of Charleston   13

Chapter 4   A Broken Life   17

Chapter 5   Kevin   21

Chapter 6   Carrie   25

Chapter 7   Airlifted   29

Chapter 8   Moving On—September 2011   35

Chapter 9   Just Another Day   41

Chapter 10   Conquering Defeat   45

Chapter 11   A Sense of Humor, Positive Attitude, and Determination   51

Chapter 12   One Step at a Time   59

Chapter 13   No Regrets   67

Chapter 14   Change   75

PART II   **A ROSE, AN ANCHOR, AND A COMPASS**   **79**

Chapter 15   Carrie   81

Chapter 16   Matt   89
Chapter 17   Paul   95
Chapter 18   Grandpa David and Nan   101
Chapter 19   Aunt Lori   105

PART III   **DETERMINATION**   **109**
Chapter 20   Meg's View of Therapy   111
Chapter 21   Life Is Good   117
Chapter 22   Once a Sailor, Always a Sailor   121
Chapter 23   I'm Good   125

PART IV   **A BEACON OF STRENGTH**   **129**
Chapter 24   Putting Life in Perspective   131
Chapter 25   Coach Mike   147
Chapter 26   Meg   151

PART V   **LIFE GOES ON**   **159**
Chapter 27   What If?   161
Chapter 28   We're Good   169

PART VI   **HELPFUL RESOURCES**   **171**
About the Author   175
Notes   177

MOONDANCE
By Chris O'Brien

Moondance is a Swann 44.
A sailboat designed for open-ocean racing.
She thrives in strong wind and rough seas.
She has no problem being on her own in the open ocean.
Carefully crafted,
She handles any hardships she may face.
She is a rock-solid ship,
Decorated with a dark blue hull,
Striped with a thin gold line on her sides.
Distinguishable from any other boat on the sea,
She is constructed of solid teak wood.
With a deck battered and beaten,
She has endured.
Scars on the pearl white mast show
She will never give up, can always be repaired.
She dances under the moon,
Illuminating the dark skies around her.
She is a boat.
I am *Moondance*.

Nearly Drowning

Meg 1968

———

My heart pounded. Terrible thoughts rushed through my head as fear took over my entire body. At only six years old, this life-altering event rocked my world. On this beautiful sunny day at Noroton Yacht Club, the sounds of summer echoed: kids laughing and splashing in the water, sail stays clanging together, instructors calling out, and lifeguard whistles blowing as the children headed out of the harbor on their sailboats for lessons. Inside the harbor, two large docks sat attached by a long, low, skinny dock. It was my day for swimming lessons instead of sailing class.

From the time I could walk, I loved the water and was a natural swimmer. On that day, however, my life was rattled. My swim instructor was teaching a group of six-year-olds, including myself, how to tread water and then float without sinking underwater, skills every sailor is required to master. I looked up at the blue sky while my body floated and saltwater kissed my face.

My eyes closed, and I had drifted off into my own little world of solitude when suddenly darkness surrounded me. My body tensed as I became alert. In confusion, I flapped my arms only to be scratched by barnacles. Trapped, I tried to inhale small bits of air between the water and the dock, but it wasn't enough.

With no pockets of air, panic rose through my lungs making them feel heavy. My mind played games. I knew someone would find me, but as I lost strength I thought about never taking another a breath, about the darkness and dying. My body became limp. I felt myself drifting into another world. There was a point when I just gave into the exhaustion, letting go, saying goodbye. Suddenly, I felt the strong hands of a lifeguard reaching for me, pulling me into his grasp, lifting me out of the water, and carrying me to safety.

This traumatic event scarred my early life. As a result, claustrophobia became my enemy. I struggled with small enclosed places like elevators and even big crowded spaces. The panicked feeling would come back to me even in situations when I wasn't in danger. Now, as an adult, my fears have lessened so that I can reason with myself and not let panic take over. Through determination, I did not let this near-drowning experience inhibit my love for swimming, sailing, and other water sports. Sometimes life throws us curve balls, but these experiences are what make us who we are today.

While no one can completely comprehend how Chris felt at the time of his accident and the impact it has had on his life now as a quadriplegic, I wanted Chris to share *his* story, what he has endured, the strength and determination he brings to each day to walk again and face any fears that may hold him back. Chris has said, "The doctors told me I would never use my arms again. I can use my arms. The doctors told me I would never feel my legs or move them again. I can feel them, and I am beginning to have movement. The doctors told me I would never walk again. But I *will* walk again in this lifetime."

Chris's story is one of courage, faith, hope, and determination. Anyone who reads his story will find encouragement in times of adversity.

PART I

CHOOSING LIFE

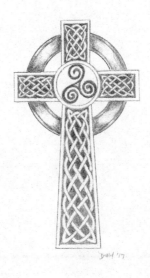

PART I

CHOOSING LIFE

CHAPTER 1

God's Plan

―――――

You have to accept whatever comes, and the important thing is
that you meet it with courage and the best you have to give.
—ELEANOR ROOSEVELT[1]

I magine four young men ages twenty-one to twenty-four, all quadriplegics, sitting at an outdoor café with their mom, sister, and a few friends. We've all been brought together from different places because of these boys and their tragic accidents. People enjoying their meals turn their heads and stare slightly, some with perplexed looks and saddened expressions at seeing these young men being spoon-fed by their mother or sister, their beer steins brought to their mouths by others' hands like they were babies being fed a bottle. But the young men are all laughing and telling stories, including those of the accidents that changed their lives forever.

Instead of being mired in regret, they look at their lives as gifts and wouldn't give up the relationships with people they've met who are now friends and part of a support system. I have known Chris

O'Brien since he was about five years old, running around playing with his brother and my boys. At age twenty-five, Chris has been a quadriplegic for six years since he innocently dove into a wave in the waters of Block Island only to hit a sandbar head first. According to the American Academy of Orthopedic Surgeons, Chris is one of eighteen hundred or more spinal cord injuries (SCIs) that result from diving accidents every year.

Growing up Chris was always polite, friendly, tall for his age, and strikingly handsome with his sandy blond hair and deep brown eyes. He spent many summer days at Pinewood Lake in Trumbull, Connecticut with my boys, Billy and Peter, his brother Matt, and a pile more. When I say a pile, I really mean it. Sometimes there would be dozens of suntanned children—mostly boys—running around without a care in the world. The moms sat in the "circle" as it was called by other members not a part of our group, while the kids swam out to the dock, played in the sand, came to us when they were hungry, and ran off again.

Our circle shared common beliefs on raising kids. Each one of us felt obligated to watch each other's kids, to help and support them when needed, which continued on into their adult years. We laughed, told stories, read magazines, shared recipes, swam with the kids, and created memories and lifelong friendships. Sometimes mornings would turn into afternoons, which would then turn into evenings on the beach. As the early evening arrived, the sky would give an orange glow that reflected off the water. A calmness took over the lake water, and the beach would empty. As the kids slowed down, they often played in the sand or sat on their towels and played cards while we moms opened some wine and continued on without a care in the world.

There was something extraordinary about those days that leaves me wishing for them back at times. Sometimes our husbands would join us, and once it was dark they would help us carry our sun-kissed, exhausted children home to a bath and bedtime so we could do it all over again the next day.

Life was good, really good. The friendships among the kids and us moms have been maintained but are different now. There were years when I didn't see Chris at all except for the holiday get-together, but I have always maintained a connection with his life in various ways. At different times, I coached him on a swim team, tutored him in writing, shared sailing stories, and lived vicariously through him when he became an avid sailor.

I think back on my life and the events that allow me to relate to Chris's story and give me the wherewithal to share it. From the time I was six years old, I spent my summers on sailboats. My dad, also a lifelong sailor, would take Mom, my two sisters, and I on overnights from Long Island Sound up to Hamburg Cove and then to Mystic, Connecticut. I have vivid memories of waking up early to set sail with my dad when it was so peaceful and calm, and later, sailing into a storm with him teasing us, "We're lost at sea." My mom would huddle with my sisters below deck while my dad and I giggled at his taunting.

From small crafts to big boats, I learned how to rig a boat, tie a bowline knot, read the wind, set and fly a spinnaker, and race during calm winds or no winds or squalls that hit Long Island Sound without warning. After graduating from the University of Vermont, I joined Noroton Yacht Club in Darien, Connecticut, where I had grown up sailing. Then a junior member, I spent Saturdays and Sundays crewing. I was an avid sailor until one winter I had a ski fall, leaving me unable to ski for the rest of the season. When sailing season rolled around again, despite my efforts, I just couldn't sail. I was in too much pain, and the discs in my lower spine were pressing on nerves, causing a drop foot.

In July 1989, I ended up in the hospital for a spinal surgery at L 4-5. My boyfriend, whom I sailed with every weekend and actually *taught* how to sail, couldn't handle the situation. Our J24 skipper and crew had referred to us as "Barbie and Ken," but perhaps we weren't really in love—just in love with sailing together. The turn of events and my being out of commission told the truth. We were nothing if we couldn't sail or ski together. We broke up, I had major back surgery, and got laid off from my job, all within weeks of each other. Life was not good. I felt lost and lonely and struggled with choosing life. I was that depressed.

Eleanor Roosevelt once said, "All that you go through here has some value. There must be a reason for it."[2] I am now able to look back on that time in my life and see that God had a plan for me, and it wasn't to be with my previous boyfriend, living a pretty wild life of partying with sailor friends late into the night, and not taking care of myself. A few days before my surgery, a friend from college invited me out to dinner with her husband, their neighbors, and their friend Brian. Brian was single, always hanging out with my friend's neighbors. I was single and always hanging out with my friend and her husband. Being in so much pain, I was in no mood for this dinner. But my friend, Ilene, encouraged me to go out with them.

As it turned out, the six of us had a nice lobster dinner on the harbor with lots of laughs that took my mind away from the pain. A few weeks later, when Brian heard about my surgery, he left an annual family vacation on Cape Cod to visit me in the hospital. From then on, he was by my side, helping me heal. I couldn't understand why Brian would do that when a boyfriend of two years didn't have the decency to visit or even send a card. Some people just can't face change. To this day Brian says that it was God's way of slowing me down so he could catch me.

So, while we don't always see clearly the reasons for events that happen in our lives, eventually the plan is revealed to us. I would go on to have three more major spinal surgeries with Brian supporting me. While my racing days are over and that adventure is a ship of the past, I am thankful. Where would I be today? I'm not sure, but I know I am in a better place.

CHAPTER 2

Chris

Be Not Afraid

━━━

I go before you always. Come follow me and I will give
you rest. If you pass through raging waters in the sea,
you shall not drown.[3]

As a teenager, I was terrified of the ocean and its vast expanse—the unknown waters that sometimes raged and sometimes calmed. Since fear is not my friend, I chose to conquer it by learning how to sail. At the age of fifteen, I started sailing on C-420s at Black Rock Yacht Club in Bridgeport, where I also swam competitively on their summer team. I became interested in big boats and started Junior Big Boat Sailing (JBBS). Sailing on J120s with peers, a few of the instructors, and the owners of the boats, we'd practice then race in the evening races on Long Island Sound. The following summer, there were so many junior racers that I began sailing solely on a Swann 44 called *Moondance*, owned by Cliff Crowley, who was integral in teaching me serious sailing skills.

At the end of the summer Cliff asked me to sail in the 75th Anniversary of the Vineyard Race over Labor Day weekend. First begun in 1932, the Vineyard Race is a classic American yachting event: a 238-mile course stretching from Shippan Point, in Stamford, Connecticut, past Block Island, and onto the entrance to Buzzard's Bay, to return leaving Block Island to starboard and finishing in Stamford Harbor. Sailors who are successful at the challenges of the race credit local knowledge of these tricky waters and a good deal of luck.[4] Sailing this race meant missing a few days of school, which my parents thankfully agreed to. As it turned out, it was literally a once-in-a-lifetime experience for me.

The following summer after my senior year in high school, I was licensed to teach sailing at Longshore Sailing School in Westport, Connecticut, and also continued sailing big boats in the evenings. One night my Aunt Lori, who grew up sailing every summer, came over for dinner. When I arrived home all excited from an evening of sailing, she looked me in the eyes and said, "Oh my gosh, Chris. You're hooked. You've got the sailing bug." *Moondance* had been tossed up on the rocks and wrecked by a storm, so Cliff gave me the number of a few friends, Colin and John in City Island, New York. It was then that I wrote the poem about *Moondance*, not realizing at the time it would be a metaphor for my own life. And so it was that I would leave Longshore, sometimes early, for City Island to sail in the Wednesday night series and then drive home late Wednesday night to go to work in the morning.

One day my boss took me aside and said I couldn't leave work early anymore. However, when I explained that I was crewing with Colin on a well-known J29 named *Hustler*, my boss made the connection that I was sailing with his longtime friend. Colin had been raving over this new kid, *me*, who was a talented young sailor with huge potential. Sometimes things are just meant to be. From then on, whenever I left work early, my boss would simply smile and wish me luck.

The sailing world opened up so many opportunities. I was asked to sail a boat with Colin to Newport for a captain who would be sailing in the Bermuda Race. Leaving Port Washington at four in the afternoon on a sunny, 85-degree summer day, we started out sailing in the calm waters of the harbor, but once out of the harbor—and into Long Island Sound—the winds picked up to about 30 knots. At one point a gust took the boat, and we almost capsized—quite a harrowing experience. That night, the temperature dropped to a chilling 45 degrees.

Sailors know that weather can fluctuate and is very unpredictable, so being prepared as we were with life jackets, foul weather gear, wool socks, and warm clothes can be a lifesaver. Colin and I had planned to take shifts sailing the boat through the night, but with the winds picking up at about 2 a.m. and a lot of boat traffic with ferries and barges, we needed all hands and eyes on deck. I realized this when at one point, as I was sailing this 40-foot yacht by myself while Colin slept below, I had to quickly change course when a tugboat crossed our path. As I came about, handling the jib and the mainsail by myself instead of with several crew members, I was scared but exhilarated at the same time. Colin felt the abrupt shift in direction of the boat and quickly joined me on deck. From then on, both of us were up on deck until arriving in Newport, Rhode Island, beaten up and weary.

A few hours before entering Newport Harbor, the most beautiful sunrise came across the horizon. The Narragansett Bay was tranquil and welcoming. After a long night, we docked the boat, cleaned the deck of the salt spray, furled the sails, and then drove back to City Island in a rental car. After leaving Newport at about 10 a.m., we stopped for a large cup of coffee and the most delicious biscuit with sausage and gravy for breakfast. Colin and I were so tired that we relished every bite in silence.

Torrential rain poured down on the ride home. I was committed to racing that night, but I was physically exhausted. My mind went back and forth thinking about whether I wanted to back out at the last minute. This may sound silly, but I called my mom to ask if it was okay. She said, "Absolutely not, Christopher. You have school, and you haven't been home in forty-eight hours," which was exactly what I had hoped she'd say. Even back then, my mom and I had a unique relationship. She could read my feelings, and I knew exactly what she was going to say. At that time in my life, I had no idea how strong our mother-son bond would be in the years to come.

CHAPTER 3

Swimming at the College of Charleston

Winners never quit, and quitters never win.
—VINCE LOMBARDI[5]

I had been in touch with the head sailing coach at the College of Charleston and sent my resume to him upon being accepted to the C of C. The coach had given me a verbal acceptance to sail 420s with the team, so I was pumped to meet him in the summer before freshman year. When my parents and I went to visit, the coach saw that I was six-foot-four and told me I was too tall to sail for him. In my anger at his response—after all my height was on my original resume—I sent him my resume again with a curt note saying, "You could have told me that over the phone."

Instantly, I looked up the swim coach's phone number and name. I called him, and surprisingly he picked up the phone right away. Coach Bruce said to meet him at his office on the pool deck. At first

I was ambivalent because I was done with swimming. With his deep voice, he told me I could be a walk-on. Literally, my plans changed within ten minutes. Within days, I was getting emails about captain's practices and schedules, and I thought, *I'm not sure I really want to swim.* The whole turn of events came about so quickly. Initially, when I visited C of C, I didn't love the college, but when I learned about the sailing program, I decided to attend. Now I would begin at the College of Charleston as a walk-on to the swim team. I ended up swimming the best race of my career my freshman year.

Through the fall of 2010, I hated, hated, HATED swim practice. I was working to improve my times, but I was not where I needed to be to compete with the team. My days were driven by practice and lifting, with very little time for academics or fun. Christmas break came in early December, and while most people were heading back home for the holidays, I was at school until December 22 with double practices each day, which took two weeks away from being at home.

This was so hard. I love being home with my family and friends, especially during the holidays, but I was home for only five days and then it was off to Miami with three practices every day. I did not want to go back to continue swimming and begged my parents to let me quit, but they said, "You are not a quitter, Chris," and I knew I had to at least finish the year out. Looking back, I'm so thankful for that, because it was after the break that my times improved. Instead of being last, I was winning races.

The trip to Miami was painful. I got into a lot of arguments with a couple of teammates. My New England upbringing was very different from that of the Southern guys. I didn't see eye-to-eye with a few of the guys, and one night I just lost it. I slammed my fist down on the table, sending dishes and drinks to the ground, and hollered at a teammate that he'd better quit making comments about people and their beliefs. I surprised myself, and even my coach went silent. Another night at a bar, when we weren't supposed to be out, the same teammate made me so mad I took a swing at him, surprising both of us. After that we reconciled some differences and acted more like teammates.

Hard work finally paid off when I went from 51 seconds in my 100-yard freestyle to 47.6 in the Coastal Collegiate Swimming Association (CCSA) Conference Championship in April 2011, where I took first place in my heat. My body was in rhythm with the water, my stroke strong and my kick streamlined. The days of practicing my kick for endless hours had finally come together, and I felt it completely. The moment I touched the wall, I heard my teammates screaming out my name and I knew. After all that hard work and determination, I had won the race. Then, unknowingly at the time, I swam the very last 50-yard freestyle race of my life in 21.9 seconds, a huge leap from when I first arrived at C of C. My best buddy Greg, who had been practicing his kick with me day in and day out, high-fived me and gave me a brotherly hug and pat on the back. Really, if it hadn't been for him, I might have given up. He always gave me the drive to keep at it. What a victory it was for me and my team. It was after my victory that I decided to celebrate and get the tattoo on my left inner bicep—a Gaelic cross, now very symbolic of my life.

The following year, my team won the CCSA Conference in my name, but physically I was not there. I remember well my spring coach, Bora, from Turkey. He had ripped me apart when I wasn't kicking right and pushed me hard to stay focused and determined. In one way or another, his tough coaching style prepared me for where I am today. Today, my long board is hanging on his office wall in memory of how far I had come.

When I think back to my younger days of swimming and my success at the C of C, my high school coach comes to mind. Coach Mike looked out for me and told me that I had huge potential and would swim in college. Being a teenager, I took his words of encouragement lightly at first, but over the years they became intrinsic.

CHAPTER 4

A Broken Life

———

The world breaks everyone, but afterward
many are strong in the broken places.
—**ERNEST HEMINGWAY** [6]

My freshman year of college was over, and my close friends from high school were all home to begin summer vacation jobs in a few days. My buddies Kevin, Pat, and I decided to head to Block Island, Rhode Island, for a day on the beach. We hopped on the ferry from New London, Connecticut, with our beach towels, coolers filled with food and drinks, and a volleyball. Within ninety minutes we were on the beach on this 95-degree, blue-sky day, and the water was just right for swimming. Of course, we planned on meeting some people, maybe even some girls. What more could we ask for. It was going to be a perfect day.

As we had planned, we met a lot of people that day and even bumped into a few we knew from home. Block Island has seventeen miles of white sandy beaches to explore, and our plan was to see them all and end up at Mansion Beach. All day we ran around from one part of the beach to another, reveling in our teenage freedom, playing volleyball and just hanging out, laughing and living life. We never did make it to Mansion Beach. The mood of the day changed like the blink of an eye. At 5 p.m., my mom called to check in. Just a quick hello and when will you be home. We planned to take a 7 p.m. ferry after the next volleyball game and a quick swim. I clicked off my cell phone, finished a friendly but aggressive volleyball game, and decided to go for the last swim of the day. The waves had gotten bigger and stronger as the day went on, and the tide was high.

"I'll race you to the buoy," Kevin hollered as he charged into the water. After giving Kevin a fifteen-second head start because he's not a strong swimmer, I ran and took my usual swimmer's dive into one of the approaching waves. At that moment, my life changed forever. Kevin later said he made it to the buoy, looked back, and I was not there.

A girl we'd been hanging out with was swimming out to him, yelling frantically, "There's a problem with Chris!" In a panic, Kevin swam back to shore against the waves as fast as he could to find me floating in the water. Pat was about to join in Kevin's challenge when he saw me lying face down on top of the water. It had all happened so fast. My hands had hit first and now dangled beside me, my ears rang, my body felt numb and fuzzy, and I was unable to move. It must have been a sandbar brought in with the tide. I clearly saw the ripples in the sand below me. Paralyzed, my body was frozen in place.

Being a swimmer my whole life, I could hold my breath for long periods of time and was able to keep myself afloat. Immediately, I knew my situation was bad. My heart was racing, but for some reason I did not panic. Pat pulled me out of the water with all his strength and turned me over. By then a nervous crowd had formed. Lying there surrounded by a circle of people, all eyes on me, I was for a moment right there with the crowd, looking at myself from above. It was a surreal moment in time as though my soul had left my body so that I could take in what was happening.

As soon as Kevin got to me, he busted through the crowd, stumbling on his words and crying out, "What's going on? What happened?"

"I'm o...kay, but can...can't feel any...thing," I stuttered.

Kevin and Pat clearly knew I wasn't okay, that I needed medical attention immediately. I lay there paralyzed, unable to move my body. Amazingly, there were several doctors on the beach who rushed to my rescue. The lifeguards jumped into survival mode, helped the doctors, put a collar around my neck, and slowly moved me onto a board with help from Kevin and Pat. My head hung slightly off the top of the board, and it hurt like hell. Together they lifted me onto an ATV, and the guards drove me to the Emergency Care Center down the beach. Since there was no room on the ATV, a woman in the crowd said she'd give Kevin and Pat a ride. They jumped in her red Volkswagen and sped toward the Emergency Care Center, where I was immediately put on a bed with an IV as the medical team made plans to have me airlifted to either Rhode Island Hospital or Hartford Medical.

CHAPTER 5

Kevin

Without friends no one would choose to live.
—ARISTOTLE [7]

C hris was fading in and out. I didn't want to leave his side, but I had to call his mom, Carrie. First I called Matt, Chris's younger brother, to get her cell phone number, and I told Matt there had been an accident. Matt was really upset, but I played it down, despite the cracking in my voice, saying he was going to be okay. When I finally called Mrs. O'Brien, I couldn't find the words to speak. Too shaken up and emotional, I handed the phone to Pat.

Mrs. O'Brien had a lucrative, full-time job with Macy's in Fine Jewelry, and she was in the car with a cosmetics manager when she got my devastating call. She was on the way home from an out-of-town business meeting and had talked to Chris just fifteen minutes earlier. Pat's voice was calm on the phone, despite his being very distraught, as he told her what had happened. A nurse on duty told Mrs. O'Brien it was urgent that Chris be airlifted; which hospital would she prefer,

21

Hartford, Connecticut, or Providence, Rhode Island? Hearing this, Chris imagined his mom on the other end of the phone, terrified but matter-of-fact and strong. "Just get him to the nearest hospital," she said.

We waited for two very long hours for the helicopter. During that time, I tried to make Chris laugh and sing songs with me despite being short of breath. I took his effort as a positive sign. Chris was taken by ambulance to a middle school where the helicopter could land. When the transport finally arrived, I hollered to the medical people on board over the sound of the propellers, "I need to go with Chris!"

Over the commotion of the helicopter, someone yelled back, "I'm sorry, kid, there's no room. You can't come on board."

Devastation washed over me as I watched Chris be airlifted. Standing desperately below the helicopter, its propellers spinning around like the panic I felt, I watched it fly off into the darkening sky, leaving me behind, tears welling up in my eyes until I could hold them no longer. I stood there and sobbed with my whole body shaking uncontrollably. Equally distraught, Pat put a hand on my shoulder and said, "Deep breath, Kevin. Deep breath. We have to keep it together for Chris."

Chris was taken to Rhode Island Hospital, where his fate would be determined. In an instant, our day had ended in a way we never could have imagined. The Block Island ferry was held for us. Pat and I boarded and sat in a heavy silence, agonizing over the day's events on the trip to New London, where my mom would pick us up and drive us directly to Rhode Island Hospital.

My life changed that day. I changed that day. Chris changed that day. My best friend was now a quadriplegic, and I felt partially responsible. If we hadn't decided to race into the water, would this even have happened? People would tell me that it wasn't my fault that it could have happened to anyone. It's taken me a long time to start believing that and to not feel at fault. From that day on, I would be there for Chris no matter what.

After the accident, I was at the hospital every day and brought friends up every Friday to hang out. In typical guy fashion, we'd act like nothing happened. We'd play music, joke around, have conversations, but not about the accident. We simply ignored the situation. It was about being normal together, like nothing ever happened—despite knowing perfectly well that a situation did indeed exist with lots of unknown questions and answers to follow.

It came time for me to go back to college in mid-August. The car was packed, and I planned to head out the next day. That night I tossed and turned thinking about Chris, and I knew I just couldn't leave. It was too far away. I couldn't imagine not being there for Chris. In the morning, not knowing whether my parents would listen, I had a talk with my dad. Freshman year at Albion College in Michigan was under my belt. My new plan was to take classes locally instead of going back to Albion. My dad, who was always saying education comes first, was silenced by my words. After thinking for what seemed like forever, he agreed, called Eastern Connecticut State University, explained the situation, and got me admitted immediately.

Relief poured over me as I realized I didn't have to leave Chris, for now. I could take classes, but also be there as much as possible when Chris came home from Rhode Island. When he began treatment at Gaylord in Connecticut, I helped with his pool therapy, home therapy, and then therapy at Life Design in Shelton. I would set up sprints for us with cones, Chris in his chair and me running. I used my conditioning for lacrosse as a means to help Chris get stronger. A full year later in August 2012, I returned to Albion to finish my undergraduate degree and play fall ball. Chris was in a good place when I finally left for school. He was heading to Shepherd Center in Atlanta, where he would get therapy at one of the best facilities for spinal cord injury. It was time for me to go back to Albion and live my life as originally planned. Despite Chris encouraging me to go, I still felt a pang of guilt about leaving him behind.

Anytime I come back for a break or holiday, the first thing on my list of things to do is to visit Chris. He is always upbeat and optimistic, every time I see him. His hard work and determination are evident by his improved strength. Hanging out with Chris and his family is always comforting. It's like old times when I walk in the door and see Chris working on physical therapy or school work, and Mrs. O'Brien cooking up something delicious to eat for family and friends who stop by. In 2014, I graduated from Albion with a mass media marketing degree, and I am now working in sales in Stamford, Connecticut, while living in Trumbull, so visiting Chris is a regular occurrence. Getting Chris in and out of the car, taking care of some of his needs, taking him to the movies, out to a bar, or to the Two Roads Brewery, where we can hang out and taste IPAs, are all significant pieces of my life now.

Our friendship has changed as I feel the need to take care of Chris. On the other hand, our friendship is unchanged, because Chris is the same person inside as he was before the accident. He still has a sense of humor and loves to rattle off what he calls "useless knowledge." He is still the one person I turn to for advice. He is still the same determined Chris O'Brien I have known since middle school.

CHAPTER 6

Carrie

———

God could not be everywhere, and therefore He made mothers. [8]

A mom's worst nightmare is a phone call about her son being in an accident of any kind, let alone one of this magnitude. When I received the call from Chris's friend Pat, I was in disbelief, shock actually. My eighteen-year-old son Chris had been in a serious accident and was being airlifted to either Hartford Medical in Connecticut or Rhode Island Hospital in Providence. My first reaction was to cry, but I pulled myself together and gave directions for Chris to be airlifted to the nearest Intensive Care Unit, which was Rhode Island Hospital.

I had spoken to Chris only one hour earlier. I was thinking, *There is no way this could have happened.* He and his buddies were to take the next ferry home. Chris had been grounded for having people over while Paul and I were away, but we let him go to Block Island with his friends with the understanding that he still owed us. Now I was feeling regret and wishing I hadn't let Chris go with his friends. The words "He can't move...paralyzed" rang in my head as I drove home hurriedly from my business meeting back to Connecticut to meet my husband, Paul. We would meet and head directly to Providence to be with Chris.

We made the drive to Providence in complete silence. Paul tried to beat the horrendous evening traffic by getting off the highway onto back roads that wound up putting us an hour behind schedule. I held back my frustration by taking deep breaths and not saying what I was thinking. Otherwise, I might have fallen apart at the seams. What we both didn't know at the time was that Chris's situation would be life altering for him, for us, and for our entire family.

We finally arrived at Rhode Island Hospital at 9:30 p.m. Chris was in the emergency room, strapped to a board with a collar around his neck. He couldn't turn to look at me, but stared straight up at the ceiling, his eyes worried. The first step would be some tests, including an MRI, and then the doctors would drill the halo into Chris's skull to keep his spine and neck stable. The doctors were examining Chris when I heard one say lightly, "Nice tattoo." I turned to look at Chris and saw a Gaelic cross on his left bicep.

"Christopher, what were you thinking?" I said firmly, even though it seemed minor compared to what had just happened to him. Chris had gotten the tattoo in February after finishing up the winter season of swimming. He had been discreet and hidden it from us when he came home for his grandmother's funeral in April and then all summer, knowing that we would not have approved. I remembered a conversation back in January when Chris asked his dad if he could get a tattoo. Like most dads, Paul said, "Ask your mother," which is when Chris knew if he asked me, he'd never get the tattoo.

Chris was always in the water at pool parties or any event at the beach. It struck me as odd for Chris not to take off his shirt and swim at a family pool party. He simply said, in a convincing manner, that he was tired of swimming. Just before the accident, his friends asked him what his parents thought of the tattoo. He told them we didn't know yet, not realizing that we'd know all too soon—but not in the way he had intended. Chris chose a Gaelic cross because it represents the "God of Water." How ironic it seems now that Chris was severely injured in the water, but also saved. As I thought deeper about Chris's tattoo and learned more about its meaning, I realized that this tattoo truly symbolizes Chris's faith, hope, and determination to walk again.

Helen Keller once said, "Faith is the strength by which a shattered world shall emerge into the light."[9] Chris's faith runs deep, and even though his world has been shattered, he is still the same Chris. He is still the same boy I gave birth to. He has the same will and drive he did growing up, and I know that determination is what will help him achieve his goal of walking again.

CHAPTER 7

Airlifted

No one takes my life away from me. I give it up of my own free
will. I have the right to give it up, and I have the right to take it
back. This is what my Father has commanded me to do.

(JOHN 10:18 GNB)

I remember getting lifted onto the helicopter, the fierceness of the wind, then taking off. There was a pilot and a few other people on the helicopter. I must have lost consciousness because the next thing I knew I was on the tarmac, the wind and the noise very startling to me. My first memory of being in the hospital emergency room was being absolutely freezing and throwing up, most likely due to spinal shock. The spinal cord goes into shock for a period of time after an injury like mine. My reflexes, movements, and feelings below the injury were absent. The doctors didn't tell me anything, but I knew that my prognosis couldn't be good.

After an MRI, the doctors screwed a halo brace onto my head to mobilize my neck and body. The residual sand on my body irritated my skin quickly and resulted in bedsores and a lot of discomfort. Doctors manually pulled my spine apart to relieve the pressure on my spinal column. The sounds of instruments screwing the halo to my head and the painful pulling apart of my spine were barbaric. I didn't know this at the time, but the halo brace would not be removed until August 10, 2011, almost a month after the accident.

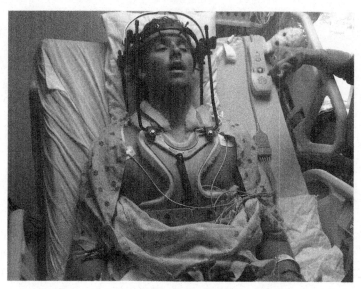

Chris in the halo brace at Rhode Island Hospital

A halo brace is a brace used to prevent your neck and head from moving. It keeps your neck in the correct position. This allows your injured spinal column and the ligaments to heal. It also helps support your neck muscles. This brace keeps your neck from moving forward, bending backward, and your head from turning. Staying in bed may cause many pressure sores, blood clots, and other health problems. The halo brace lets you get out of bed and start moving sooner after your injury.[10]

By the next day, friends and family members surrounded my hospital bedside. Of course, Kevin and Pat were there from the night before. All were stunned and in disbelief. I could read their thoughts and feel their empathy from the looks on their faces, but I did not want them to feel sorry for me. Monsignor Shea, from St. Catherine of Siena Church where I had been very involved, came in the room wearing his clerical dress to visit and give me "The Anointing of the Sick." I'd never seen him outside of church dressed that way, and my first response was, "Monsignor, am I dying or something?"

He responded with his Irish chuckle, "No, Chris, you are not dying, you are still very much alive." I would think about his words every day.

A flurry of activity surrounded me—doctors and nurses coming in and out, monitors beeping, needles getting stuck into my arm. My neck was broken at the C4-C5 level and my vertebrae had shattered into hundreds of pieces due to the impact. My spinal cord was bruised not severed; however, I was now considered a quadriplegic, or tetraplegic.

Quadriplegia is defined in different ways depending on the level of injury to the spinal cord.[11] The degree of injury to the cellular structures of the spinal cord is very important. A complete severing of the spinal cord will result in complete loss of function from that spinal segment down. A partial severing or even bruising or swelling of the spinal cord results in varying degrees of mixed function and paralysis. A common misconception with quadriplegia is that the victim cannot move legs, arms, or control any of the major bodily functions; this is often not the case. Some quadriplegic individuals can walk and use their hands as though they did not have a spinal cord injury, while others may use wheelchairs although they may still have function in their arms and mild finger movement. This is dependent on the degree of damage done to the spinal cord.[12]

Spinal cord injuries are classified by the American Spinal Cord Injury Association based on functional impairment and graded from A to D, with A being most severe. My injury is classified as "C Incomplete," which means that I have motor function and feeling below the level of injury, and more than half of the muscles below the neurological level have a muscle grade of 3. Grade 3 means that I can move a muscle against gravity. For example, I can do a bicep curl without added weight.

Within a few weeks I was out of ICU and moved to Step Down. Doctors believed I was strong enough for a procedure and performed a spinal surgery. My C4 vertebrae and disc were removed and replaced with a titanium plate and screws, and my C5 disc was taken out and replaced with a titanium cage packed with bone that would eventually fuse together. This would relieve some of the pain and discomfort, stabilize the spinal column, and prevent more injury to the area, but it would not change my diagnosis. Damage to C4-C5 meant that my shoulder muscles, neck, front arm muscles, and wrist muscles were dramatically impaired.

While the surgery went well, I spent my days lying down in bed and ended up with pneumonia. A PA had just checked me out and said my lungs sounded clear. But later, when I was rolled over onto my side, I couldn't catch my breath. I felt like I was drowning all over again, but unlike Block Island, when I knew how to hold my breath, I didn't know what to do, and this time I panicked. An X-ray technician scurried into the room and took an X-ray, which showed fluid in my lungs, confirming that I did indeed have pneumonia. People with spinal cord injuries are one hundred fifty times more likely to die from pneumonia than other causes, at any time after their injury.[13]

The doctors gave me two options: they could do a tracheotomy or insert a tube into my lungs to vacuum out the fluid. A tracheotomy or a tracheostomy is a temporary or permanent opening surgically created through the neck into the trachea (windpipe) to allow direct access to the breathing tube; it's commonly done in an operating room under general anesthesia. A tube is usually placed through this opening to provide an airway and to remove secretions from the lungs. Breathing is done through the tracheostomy tube rather than through the nose and mouth.[14]

There was no way I was letting anyone cut a hole in my neck and insert tubes to help me breathe, even if it was temporary. Several people I met later during therapy had tracheostomies and had to learn how to talk again. So the medical team inserted tubes up my nose and down the back of my throat. A vacuum then cleaned out the fluid, which had the consistency of peanut butter. This regimen continued for two and a half days. Pneumonia being very dangerous in my situation, the doctor put me on heavy doses of antibiotics. Unfortunately, antibiotics kill the probiotics in your system, which can cause other serious illnesses like clostridium difficile, known as C. Diff. This germ causes diarrhea, fever, loss of appetite, nausea, and stomach pain. In other words, my digestive tract was a mess, and so was I—literally. The diarrhea lasted for several days and would come on so fast there was no way to get me to the bathroom quickly enough. C. Diff is so contagious that I was quarantined. Doctors and nurses came into my room wearing masks and gloves, which made me feel even worse.

Meanwhile my parents had been researching rehabilitation facilities, and we had decided on RUSK in New York. I was ready to go when the C. Diff happened, and RUSK would not take me. To make things worse, Hurricane Irene hit the East Coast with full force on August 27, 2011. As the extreme weather conditions outside heightened, inside the wind was knocked out of my sails. RUSK seemed like the best opportunity for a fleeting moment, and now I was stuck in the hospital until the hurricane was over, worrying and wondering when I was going to get out of there. My mom paced the halls and waited, but she was also planning our next steps. From the beginning, we always knew when it was time—time to move on to the next place for rehabilitation.

One thing you should know about my mom is that she is a planner and can make things happen. A very significant example, and turning point for me and my family, was when one of my doctors said, "We all know Chris will never walk again."

My mom retorted, "And who told you that Chris would never walk again?" She knew it was time to find care that supported my mission, and that's exactly what she did.

CHAPTER 8

Moving On—
September 2011

The present is the ever moving shadow
that divides yesterday from tomorrow.
In that lies hope.
—FRANK LLOYD WRIGHT[15]

F inally, after more than a month at Rhode Island Hospital, I was
transferred by ambulance, strapped in and flat on my back, for
a grueling three-hour ride to Gaylord Rehabilitation Center
in Wallingford, Connecticut, where I would begin physical therapy.
Gaylord is a member of the Spaulding New England Regional Spinal
Cord Injury Center, one of just fourteen programs nationwide to be
designated as a Spinal Cord Injury Model System by the U.S. National
Institute on Disability and Rehabilitation Research (NIDRR).[16]

Gaylord had a comforting environment with very caring and
dedicated staff. It was where I would make some progress but

also realize the magnitude of my injury. At first I took some steps backward and faced challenges in my rehabilitation that I had not expected. Mom, Dad, Aunt Lori, and my grandparents, Grandpa and Nan, all took turns staying with me. There was a concern that if I needed help and no one was in the room, I'd be in trouble. My hands weren't functioning, so I couldn't even press the call button. Some plans would need to be put in place to allow me more independence. Not only was I bedridden but I couldn't urinate on my own, so a Foley catheter was inserted into my bladder to drain urine. As a result, I kept getting urinary tract infections (UTIs) and kidney infections, which meant more antibiotics. I wouldn't really know for some time how much bladder function I would have after my injury.[17]

Certain parts of the urinary system are affected by damage to the spinal cord. The kidneys will continue to filter urine from the blood, and the ureters will continue to push the urine into the bladder for storage until urination takes place. The kidneys and ureters still work because they are involuntary processes and do not require signals passed from the brain via the spinal cord.

The main process of the urinary system that is affected following a spinal cord injury is urination, or emptying the bladder on a voluntary basis. Urination requires that messages be sent to and from the brain via the spinal cord. If the spinal cord is damaged, relaxation of the sphincter muscle and contraction of the detrusor muscle may be affected, resulting in an inability to urinate properly. The sense of a full bladder may also be lost, as sensory signals from the bladder will not be able to travel to the brain through the damaged spinal cord. Different levels of injury affect different nerves which allow the bladder to function, and this is a deciding factor in choosing the right bladder management program.[18]

My calcium levels were low due to lack of weight-bearing movement. It's true what people say about being an advocate for yourself. Once the calcium levels were low, my mom went to one of the nurses and said, "We have to get Chris out of bed and help him stand so we can get his calcium levels up." As they got me up using a Hoyer, which is like a hoist, my calcium levels improved quickly.

A few weeks into my stay at Gaylord, I was tested and fitted for a "power chair," which is exactly what it sounds like. When I understood that I was not getting a "manual chair," I got very upset. It was as though no one thought I'd walk again. My ability to walk on my own was obviously my goal, and a power chair would keep me from that. People did not seem to understand that I was determined to walk again by myself. Seven months later, after much frustration and advocating for myself, I finally got the chair I wanted. Not from the state, though, as I had been promised. Thanks to the Obie Harrington-Howes Foundation, which provides financial support to people with spinal cord injuries, I would be rolling around in my brand-new swag chair, as I had planned.

By mid-October, my neck collar was removed, another step in the right direction, and by November 2011, I knew it was time to move again. This time I was going home. I hadn't been home since July 27, when my buddies and I had left on the ferry for Block Island. Our neighbor, Steve, built an entry ramp and remodeled the bathroom which made the house handicap-accessible, and a hospital bed with electrical stimulation controls was brought into the dining room, which became my bedroom.

Without the help of doctors or nurses, my family and friends learned how to care for me on their own. It was amazing how many people stepped up to help. Mom's friends, Andrea, Lori, and Amy, would come over in the mornings and evenings to get me out of bed and showered. There was no modesty involved there. I had no choice but to have help with my daily hygiene—sometimes four people at a time—which made me even more determined to claim back my independence. Therapists came to the house and worked on my shoulder mobility and arm contraction, but there was not much improvement. Some really great days kept me focused. I had been convinced that within six months I'd be walking again. But six months turned into eight months of having therapists come to the house before I would finally get accepted to Shepherd Center in Atlanta and begin therapy on August 22, 2012.

During the eight months at home, people came to support me with incredible generosity. I had previously been a volunteer firefighter with the Trumbull Center Fire Department, which is a brotherhood. Everyone looks out for each other. Michael, one of the guys, decided to hold a successful boot drive in front of Porricelli's, the local grocery store at the time. Members of the Connecticut Firefighters Pipe and Drums heard my story and sponsored me in their 8th annual fundraising event, which took place on a sunny spring afternoon in Bridgeport at Tiago's Bar and Grill, where hundreds of people came to support me. It was such an honor to be surrounded by so many people who cared and believed in me.

My aunts, Lori and Kathy O'Brien, planned a fundraiser event at Four Seasons in Bridgeport on May 4, 2012. The benefit, "Catch a Wave of Determination," raised over $100,000 toward my upcoming rehab in Atlanta. People came from all over to support me, and those who couldn't attend made significant donations. The party was a celebration of my life, and very emotional for my family, my friends, and me. Speeches were made, tears were shed, stories were told about me before my accident, and stories were told about my *determination* to walk again. The whole event was unfathomable. The money allowed me to go to Shepherd for significant rehabilitation and helped out with other medical costs already incurred.

Since the accident, my mom had to quit her job as a manager with Macy's, and insurance was only partially covering costs. The financial challenges were tremendous, and I felt bad that my parents had to endure such a burden. My accident changed the lives of numerous people whether I realized it or not.

"Music in the Grass" was another amazing fundraising event coordinated by a musician and friend of the family, Chris Mendola. Chris was inspired to put this event together when he learned of my story and my determination to walk again. Seeing these performers of all ages singing and playing music on my behalf was unbelievable. What people are willing to do for others is humbling. Imagine an outdoor festival on a beautiful summer afternoon in suburban Connecticut with food cooking on the grill, chairs and tables filled with family and friends laughing and enjoying themselves, and among them many sitting on blankets in the grass in front of an old barn with a huge backdrop of a guitar in the grass.

Music filled the yard all afternoon, T-shirts were sold, and about $50,000 was collected toward my continued rehabilitation. My experience has taught me a lot about life and how people come together in times of need. It takes a lot of determination on my part, but without the support of others, I wouldn't be where I am today. As my mom put it, "Chris Mendola was a Godsend putting this event together. We are forever grateful."

Meanwhile, my brother, who means the world to me, designed and sold T-shirts in my name. One night after a soccer game, Matt was out to dinner with our dad and came up with the idea and the logo, "Sails of Hope, Winds of Faith, Waves of Courage...Success," which expressed Matt's optimistic attitude and his desire to be by my side through thick and thin. I have no doubt that Matt was struggling inside, coping on his own, and not wanting to burden anyone with his fears and worries. It was his senior year of high school, and Matt had applied to colleges with little help from Mom, Dad, or myself, in the hopes of attending Fordham University in the fall of 2012.

Unfortunately, Matt was not accepted to Fordham but to Siena College in New York, where he decided to attend and play soccer.

Matt's disappointment was fleeting, and he accepted the plan without complaining or feeling sorry for himself. Matt's friends from soccer also decided they wanted to do something to help raise money and designed a blue bracelet saying "Chris O'Brien...Determination." Sales of the bracelets took off like wildfire. Kids of all ages were buying and wearing the bracelets, expressing their hopes for my recovery, and the money went toward my rehabilitation. I even made an appearance at Booth Hill, my elementary school, where all five hundred or so kids sported the bracelet to support me. These events and the support kept me going. I couldn't let these people down.

Before I knew it, Matt was heading off to Siena for his freshman year to study marketing and play D1 soccer. It was an emotional time for all of us. Sadly, Matt would not have Mom or me in the stands cheering him on this year as we did in the past. It was a matter of fact; our family had to divide and conquer. My mom and I were a team, and Matt and my dad were a team. My mom would continue researching and finding the best places for my rehabilitation, continue getting me to and from rehab, and be my constant caregiver, while my dad would get to as many of Matt's soccer games as possible between traveling for work and intermittent visits. Our life as a family was very different now, but despite all odds, we remained connected and supportive of each other.

CHAPTER 9

Just Another Day

One who gains strength by overcoming obstacles possesses the
only strength which can overcome adversity.
—ALBERT SCHWEITZER[19]

On August 22, 2012, I arrived at Shepherd Center in Atlanta.
That first day, I was a bit rattled when a man receiving
therapy as a quadriplegic, just like I would, died from a clot
in his leg that traveled to his lungs. I didn't ask too many questions,
but upon entering the therapy room, the atmosphere was enough
to tell me that the physical therapists felt helpless, and the patients
were facing a sad reality check for what can happen to any of us at
any time. I wondered about this stranger's family, his life, *his* story
and thought about how quickly it can all end. With this adverse, but
realistic introduction to Shepherd, I made a goal of getting to know
the people I would meet, their lives, and their stories.

Mom and I had an apartment within the campus, or Shepherd
neighborhood. The facility was walking distance, or wheeling distance

I should say, from where I had my therapy every day. There was access to the pool, weight room, adaptive machines, basketball court, and more. The lifeguards and staff would do anything to help patients, and I grew fond of many. The people staying in the apartments were there for similar reasons. We met some interesting people, to say the least. One in particular stands out to me: a girl in her late twenties who'd had a massive stroke. Not only was her left side paralyzed, but she couldn't speak clearly. When we did some therapy together, I could tell she was smart and had a positive attitude despite her bleak situation. It is one thing to be paralyzed and another to have your wits about you but not be able to communicate. She made me feel like I was in a better place.

There was also a twenty-seven-year-old man who had been a NASCAR driver. He raced in an open-wheel car, rolled the car over, and flattened it like a pancake. He coded three times but was revived, now a quadriplegic, and ended up at Shepherd after the accident. Then there was Jimmy, a forty-five-year-old man who had survived a motorcycle accident but lost his leg above the knee and had severe cervical spinal cord injury. This combined injury left him on a ventilator. He once said to my mom, "When I see Chris each day, I have to put a smile on my face to greet him." Even so, I knew he wasn't doing well, and I would engage in conversation to help *his* morale.

A day in the life at Shepherd was very physical, painful at times, and emotional too. My first day had started out emotionally hearing about the quadriplegic patient dying. I felt my mortality threatened by this close-to-home death. Otherwise, I was up and having breakfast by 8 a.m. with a peer group and an occupational therapist. Then I would work with a physical therapist for a grueling hour of mobility work like transferring myself from my chair to another chair repeatedly. From there, I'd work with Kelly, another trained exercise therapist. She'd blast music, and I'd be doing jumping jacks in my standing frame, which was really just flapping my arms. Or I'd be on a mat working on shoulder strengthening, core work, and balance.

It was tough, and it didn't end there. From 11 to 12 noon, I'd have more therapy with a different therapist. I might be rolling myself in my chair up and down the halls, which may sound easy but was incredibly challenging. I didn't have the strength then that I do now. My hands did not function the way they needed to in order to maneuver independently. I needed a lot of assistance. The muscles in my hands were so tight that I couldn't change their position from palm up to palm down. They were frozen in place. By noon, Mom and I would be back at the apartment for lunch. Sometimes my body was so physically exhausted after lunch, I didn't want to go back to Shepherd for the afternoon. I'd rally because Mom would say, "Chris, this is why we are here. Get back out there."

The afternoon consisted of occupational therapy, where I'd work on picking things up off the table, putting on a T-shirt, and other activities that would help with daily living skills. I was failing miserably for lack of arm functioning. After OT, there was a class provided by a doctor, specialist, or another person with SCI that included counseling, discussions on medical and physical issues, how to do skin checks, and sometimes peer support. After having been at home for some time, I didn't really feel like I needed this, but it was all part of the program.

There were even field trips, which I totally did not want to attend. I had been to the mall at home, out to restaurants, and out with friends. To me it was a waste of time. I wasn't too intimidated by the outside world, except for one time. My dad and I were going back to the car from a shopping mall when a girl parked in a handicap spot. I told her she shouldn't park there because it was a handicap space. She turned around, called me a "crippled asshole," and peeled out. We were in such shock, neither of us could come back with a comment as she screeched out of the parking lot at full speed.

Annoyed at first, I later realized that she was angry at life and had treated me like she might any other person, which, ironically, made me feel quite good. Despite my dad being completely disturbed by this young woman when she said she was going to "pop him," I actually had a good laugh later and chalked it up to another day's experience in my quadriplegic world.

Chapter 10

Conquering Defeat

Now is the time to start something new.
—A FORTUNE COOKIE

My therapy changed when the doctors decided my hands and arms needed "serial casting." The goal behind casting was to get the tight muscles to straighten or bend into a more natural position. My arms were wrapped in two inches of gauze and dipped into a fiber casting which would then harden. For three excruciating days, I wore the cast. It was very painful, hot, and felt heavy. I couldn't sleep, I couldn't shower, I couldn't do anything for myself. My mom was at my beck and call, which I suppose she was getting quite used to by now. She had realized that *I* was now her full-time job. After three days, the doctor cut off the cast and started the procedure all over again. My arm was turned and stretched and casted again for another three days.

Once my right arm went through the procedure three times, the same was done to my left arm three times. The whole process took five grueling weeks. Once the final casts were cut off, a "clam shell" cast was made for me to wear at night, kind of like a retainer you wear after braces. Casting of my arms and hands was one of the most difficult experiences during my stay at Shepherd, but it was also one of the most effective and productive procedures done. So effective that one of the doctors used my results in a presentation to Shepherd staff.

After two months at Shepherd, I was put through a treadmill study and qualified for a NeuroRecovery Network Study (NRN of the Christopher & Dana Reeve Foundation). I was accepted and would return to Shepherd in January 2013. Upon returning to Shepherd, I was tested again after thirty workouts on the treadmill where measurements were taken and my strength gains were recorded. I was really getting stronger: my balance, my abs, my overall strength. Unfortunately, my knee was hyperextending, which meant that when I stood up my knee extended too far back. After ninety sessions or so, they took me out of the study due to this hyperextension. For me to continue with the treadmill activities, I'd needed a knee brace, but the NRN study did not allow any extra variables. Instead, I continued in an outpatient capacity at Shepherd.

I refused to let the disappointment defeat me. There was a track around the basketball court, so I'd go up there and push myself around the track in my chair daily. I also worked out at the gym, which is where I met Jorie. Jorie would later become one of the most significant people involved in my progress both physically and mentally. Jorie was, and still is, an exercise specialist with Shepherd's "Beyond Therapy" program. Beyond Therapy works with patients and does not accept insurance, so the specialists are able to be more creative with their therapy treatments. Jorie and I would joke around. She knew about my frustration with being dismissed from the study. We became great friends, sharing a similar sense of humor, the same taste in movies, and she could make me laugh until my stomach hurt.

We hired Jorie to be my personal trainer two times per week, and she completely understood my ambitions and my determination to walk again. She pushed me to my limits, which was exactly what I needed.

One night my parents and I went out for Chinese food, and my dad's fortune cookie read, "Now is the time to try something new." It was spot-on. And try something new I did. On April 18, 2013, with my pool therapist's help, I swam with sharks at the Atlanta Aquarium Ocean Voyager Exhibit. The morning of this adventure, I had an adrenalin rush that I hadn't felt in a long time. One of the pool therapists, Michelle, was going to swim with me. She was so nervous she could hardly breathe. We made a deal, though, that if I did it, she'd do it.

First we got fitted for wetsuits and gear. Getting the wetsuit on me, let alone off, made us laugh hysterically and took about twenty minutes each time. The tank was the size of two football fields filled with about 6 million gallons of clear saltwater and had a temperature of 72 degrees, which is very cold for a quadriplegic.

We got in the tank from a platform, and Michelle held onto me as if her life depended on it. So I swam on the top of the water, facedown, floating in my wetsuit and snorkel with Michelle at one side and a trained staff member on my other. There were several 50-foot whale sharks swimming around, a few 12-foot sharks, some manta rays, hammerheads, and thousands of other fish. The whale sharks, the biggest fish species in the world, swam slowly around the tank, getting close enough to us that we could see their 4-foot mouths and their unique spotted patterns. Later, Michelle and I talked about how ironic it was that she was terrified, while I remained calm and tranquil, feeling like part of the tank itself similar to my younger years when I swam competitively.

During that time from January 2013 to July 2013, I was blessed with meeting some of the most amazing people with incredible stories—people I wouldn't have met if I hadn't been in the accident. There was an African American woman named Angela who I'd seen walking around the track regularly. One day she stopped me on the track and said, "I want to know your story. You seem happy all the time, and you seem to have it all figured out. Your smile is a gift, and your hard work commendable." I introduced myself and told her my story. "I'll pray for you," she said. "I have a lot of boys I'm praying for."

A week or so later, I saw Angela with a middle-aged man in Beyond Therapy who had a brain injury. The man was from her church, and Angela drove him to and from Shepherd for his appointments. After my mom got to know her, Angela shared her story. She had a son in the military and another son who had been doing a night bank delivery in Atlanta and was shot to death. To tell her son in the military that his brother had been shot right in his very own city did not make sense. Angela began to help boys and men who were injured in or out of the military. The last I heard, she was heading to Dubai with her church service ministry.

Not only did I meet other people, quadriplegics and paraplegics, but I met the staff at Shepherd and became very close with many. There were "the girls" as my mom called them: Kelly, Lauren, Sara, and Michelle. The girls became very protective of me and family to all of us. We took a trip to Nashville with them and had a blast listening to country bands, going to bars and restaurants, staying up late into the night, and laughing a lot like ordinary adults.

For such brilliant minds, the girls were sometimes so surprisingly silly. One evening they were waiting for us in the lobby and saw there was free orange juice and what they thought was champagne. They mixed it together and drank what they thought were mimosas, hoping to get a buzz before going out. When we arrived in the lobby, they were literally rolling around on the floor crying from laughing so hard at themselves once they learned the champagne was actually lemonade. Their laughter always got me laughing too.

When it was time to leave Shepherd in July, Lauren—who was one of the lifeguards at the therapy pool—came running to us and hollered, "We are coming to see you in Connecticut, all four of us!" And they did. In September, they arrived in Connecticut and we drove up to Boston for a few days. Despite my being a few years younger and a quadriplegic, the girls were genuine and treated me like any other person and friend. They kept their eyes on me, but they let me lead the way, not holding me back except for once when I was pushing my chair along and hit a curb. Kelly was right there to grab the back of my chair and stop it before I toppled over into the busy street. Mom became like a mother to Kelly, Lauren, Sara, and Michelle. Perhaps we knew more about their personal lives than most people do of their therapists, but their families weren't around to be part of their life experiences like we were.

CHAPTER 11

A Sense of Humor, Positive Attitude, and Determination

The most wasted of all days is one without laughter.
—E. E. CUMMINGS[20]

Approved for a Lokomat Study, and after a long stay at home in Connecticut, I returned to Shepherd in January 2014. The Lokomat allows a patient to stand and get weight-bearing activity, an essential part of strengthening and recovery from SCI. Shepherd felt like home as soon as I saw Jorie. Six months had passed since my last stay at Shepherd, but we immediately laughed with one of our inside jokes. Another PT, Katie, said to Jorie, "I haven't heard you laughing like this since Chris left." When working with Jorie at Beyond Therapy, I'd spike my hair. There was this exercise she made me do on a massage table with my face down in the hole. My hair would go into wild spikes, and Jorie called it "Hair by Jorie." She made the challenging therapy fun with word-play games and jumbles that kept me thinking less about how hard I was working. With some laughter and a sense of humor, time would fly by.

Making connections with people is a skill I learned through my family, friends, and experiences in college, and now it is one I use more than ever. New people are coming into my life every day. I figure out what people like to do, what they are interested in, passionate about, and then I research and find information so I can talk to them. My exercise specialist, Jordan, loves soccer. I was never athletically inclined other than swimming and sailing, so the only connection with soccer I had was to watch my brother, Matt, play for his teams. Since Jordan also became a friend, I started downloading statistics so I could talk intelligently about the sport and world games. As a result, soccer became a personal interest.

The Lokomat Study did not go as planned. When I was retested for the study, I failed. Before leaving Shepherd in July 2013, I was able to move my right toes on command. Upon returning in 2014, that was not the case. A research scientist working with me kept retesting me, but nothing changed, which meant I couldn't participate in the study—and it would be costly to stay at Shepherd. My first reaction was complete shock. Again, the wind was knocked out of my sails. I could hardly breathe and felt a wave of nausea rise up into my throat. I had returned to Shepherd primarily to participate in this study, and now it was over. Leaving the testing room in disbelief, I had to tell my parents this devastating news. I could hear them talking and laughing before rounding the corner, then saw them coming toward me. Shaking my head, I blurted loudly, "There's no study. I'm out." Mom's eyebrows rose, and her expression became suddenly serious.

My dad's voice boomed, "Now what? What the heck are we going to do?" He was angry and extremely frustrated since he had to head back to Connecticut without a plan for me. My mom immediately tried to figure things out while dealing with the combined emotions of all three of us. Since we had just signed a six-month lease on the apartment, we needed to find a way to make the best of the situation without incurring out-of-pocket therapy expenses.

"Let me think about this," was my mom's reaction. "Are you sure that is what you heard, Chris?" She went down to Beyond Therapy and talked with Jorie. Her thinking was if we couldn't do the day program or do the study, there was only Beyond Therapy left. Within a day, the team at Beyond Therapy made an exception, and I was accepted into the program. I felt relieved because we had a plan. Our annual $2500 flexible spending would be used to get my therapy started, but it would not sustain us for six months. I felt defeated but knew I had to stay positive, if not for myself, then for my mom.

In need of a reprieve, we decided to go visit Mom's mom and stepdad, Nan and Grandpa, in southern Georgia. Visiting them gave us both a sense of normalcy, the comforts of home, and support. Mom was able to get a break from the daily challenges of my life. Every day Grandpa would walk, and I would roll around the neighborhood to get some exercise. My daily routine continued the same as at home or at a facility. One Saturday morning when I was in the bathroom, Grandpa told Mom he'd been doing some research and asked if she had ever heard of "crowdfunding." Without my even knowing what he was up to, my Grandpa got a campaign started by Sunday morning on my behalf. He wrote up a blurb to post on Facebook about my situation, read it over with my mom, made some minor changes, and decided to go for it. This is what he wrote:

Chris O'Brien's family needs to raise funds to pay for the Beyond Therapy spinal cord program at the Shepard Center in Atlanta, Georgia.

A broken neck is a life changing event of the first magnitude. On July 27, 2011 our grandson, Chris O'Brien, did what millions of people do every day—he dove into the surf at the beach. Sadly, he didn't know there was a sand bar shortly below the surface.

His head struck at just the right angle to break his C4 and C5 vertebrae, leaving him, at 18, face-down in the water and unable to move. Luckily, friends saw something was terribly wrong and, while Chris was fully conscious, rescued him. He was airlifted to Rhode Island Hospital where a plate and two screws were attached to the damaged bones, which were then fused together. After 30 days in the ICU he was finally released and went back to his home in CT. A quadriplegic, he is unable to walk and has very limited dexterity with hands and arms.

In the last two years he has had extensive therapy in CT, NJ and GA and has made some improvement, but is still facing years of work to regain more independence (he remains totally dependent on his caregivers - his Mom and Dad - for all daily necessities and basic functions).

He has entered the Beyond Therapy program at The Shepherd Center in Atlanta, one of the top rehab facilities in the US. This is an intensive therapy regimen which has had good success with patients in Chris's condition. The challenge is that it's not covered by insurance and costs about $900/week, not including living expenses. We are looking to raise enough to get him through about 6 months, or about $20,000.

Now 21, Chris is resuming his college studies in psychology on line at the Harvard University Extension School. He has always been a very forward looking young man and his attitude has been and remains extremely positive throughout his ordeal.

Crowdfunding is exactly what it sounds like. A fundraiser for a good cause is posted on Facebook or another social media site in hopes of raising money quickly. Friends, family, friends of family, coworkers, Grandpa's graduating class from Harvard, and many others contributed to the cause. Within a week, we had $12,000. By the end of the fundraising timeframe, people had generously donated about $30,000 in all! Now I was able to continue the therapy I needed to progress to the next step. The next six months proved successful to my rehabilitation thanks to everyone who supported and believed in me.

When I returned home and resumed therapy at Gaylord, I took 1154 steps on September 17, 2014, with the help of an EXSO™, a portable, adjustable bionic exoskeleton.[21] I had been working up to 1000 steps since the beginning of September and was determined to hit 1000 before heading back to Shepherd. It was a small victory, but one that would keep me persevering through the next phase of rehabilitation.

We were back at Shepherd by the end of September and continued Beyond Therapy until Thanksgiving, when we all reunited at home for the holidays. Always filled with the aroma of delicious food, our house was a revolving door of family and friends who visited and even stayed for extended periods of time. It was around that time that someone I had met just weeks after my accident humbled me. She said meeting me had changed her life, that I motivated her to live her life better. I was touched to think that I had so impacted her life, which shows that any person in any situation, no matter how dark, can change someone else's life. All it takes is a positive attitude and determination.

Soon after that, my Trumbull High School swim coach, Mike Ferraro, asked me to be an inspirational speaker at a New Canaan YMCA event for athletes called "Gain the Winning Edge." It surprised me at first that he wanted *me* to be an "inspirational" speaker. For one, I had never spoken in front of a crowd before and was unsure about doing this. Second, I wondered if my life experience would really make a difference in their lives. But it was decided. Matt helped me put together a PowerPoint presentation. We gathered pictures of me swimming and involved in "normal" activities before the accident, and then pictures after the accident and throughout my various therapies. Since I was speaking to high school athletes, who think nothing like my tragedy will happen to them, part of my message was "work hard, but don't take anything for granted because life is fragile." Never in a million years would I have pictured myself airlifted to a hospital, fighting for my life, and then in a wheelchair fighting to walk again. I told them no matter what their life brings, they have to stay determined to reach their goals. If I was to give up now, I'd have nothing, be nothing.

Once I began speaking to the athletes, my nerves gave way to confidence. I felt their worry, their concern for my situation, and their minds wrapping around my experience, perhaps wondering if something like this could happen to them after all. No one asked questions; I don't think they knew what to ask. What I do know is that they heard my story loud and clear, and hopefully they were inspired to stay determined through thick and thin as athletes with so much lying ahead.

There is so much pressure these days in high school to do well academically, to be popular or with the "in crowd," to get into a high-ranking college, and maybe play Division 1 sports. At their age, juniors and seniors in high school, I wasn't sure where I fit in much of the time. I was friends with different groups of people but not in one particular crowd, so being part of a team was important for me. Part of my story is how hard I worked to get to the College of Charleston and swim for a Division 1 team. It didn't come easily. I worked hard, and I leaned mostly on my family, who were my support system then, as they still are today.

My closing words of encouragement to these young athletes were, "Find those people in your lives that will support you, push you, and believe in you. The rest is all about persevering and reaching goals one step at a time. That is how you stay a winner."

CHAPTER 12

One Step at a Time

Hope is the companion of power, and mother of success; for who
so hopes strongly has within him the gift of miracles.
—SAMUEL SMILES[22]

I t's an adventure every time we go to a new rehabilitation center. Our next was on February 9, 2015, when Mom and I headed to Baltimore to Kennedy Krieger Institute. We never know exactly what to expect and usually encounter a hurdle or two. Despite our initial letdown of learning I was scheduled for only three, not four weeks, Mom and I both had a good gut feeling about Kennedy Krieger.

Kennedy Krieger is a beautiful, bright, inviting environment, very inspirational the second you walk in the door, so to speak. Our instincts proved right. When we arrived the first day, we were surrounded by kids: four-year-olds who had strokes, five-year-olds with autism, ten-year-old quadriplegics. To my amazement, they were all happy. Every one of them had a bright smile on their face while working with physical therapists. My mom's first comment was, "Don't even think about being negative here. These kids are going to look up to you."

And they did. She is *always* right. One little boy named Frankie thought he was a Power Ranger. I remember those days when imagination took over reality, unlike today when I wish my imagination could take over the reality of where I am. Well, I guess that's what was so beautiful about the experience. Frankie was a Power Ranger who had a stroke at the age of four. He was in a wheelchair that gave him strength and confidence. He laughed while he made Power Ranger noises and pretended to get me with his sword. All I could think was, *What an amazing kid.* When I was four, I was busy running around my yard with the kids in my neighborhood, going to preschool, coming home to milk and cookies, having a delicious home-cooked meal with my family, and falling into bed exhausted from my day. I didn't even know what a wheelchair was, let alone a stroke. What I saw in Frankie was hope, and yet I don't think he even realized it. At age four, he gave *me* hope, which (I didn't know at the time) is the whole philosophy behind Kennedy Krieger Institute.

Kennedy Krieger was founded in 2005; the International Center for Spinal Cord Injury (ICSCI) represents something remarkable in the field of paralysis treatment: *hope.* For many years, experts held that most improvements from SCI occurred in the first six months of recovery and that improvement was impossible after two years. Rehabilitation focused mostly on teaching patients how to compensate for injuries they thought to be irreversible. The experts were wrong.

The International Center for Spinal Cord Injury (ICSCI) at Kennedy Krieger Institute was founded on the philosophy that individuals with paralysis can always hope for recovery of sensation, function, mobility, and independence, months and even years after injury. To maximize on this potential for recovery, ICSCI offers an intense, medically supervised therapy program with a unique focus on activity-based restorative therapy. ICSCI is one of the first facilities in the world to combine innovative research with a unique focus on restoration and rehabilitation for both children and adults with chronic paralysis.[23]

Every rehabilitation center I have been to since my accident has offered something different. Gaylord Hospital, Kessler Institute for Rehabilitation, Shepherd Center—they all offered me something I needed at the time but didn't even realize. Somehow when I was at Kennedy Krieger, though, it was clear why I was there. They believed that I, Christopher O'Brien, would walk again. Every day, my physical therapists would applaud me and get excited about my strength and determination. Their enthusiasm and beaming smiles kept me going. We would arrive at Kennedy Krieger at 8:45 each morning after a forty-five-minute drive to sign a form saying nothing had changed in my history since the day before. This part of their protocol annoyed me at first; however, I came to understand that it was all part of the process. Once I was in the door to therapy, I worked hard, my hardest. Some days I didn't think I could do any more, but I persevered because the therapists wouldn't let me quit. They pushed me to my limits and beyond.

When I first arrived at Kennedy Krieger, my personal goals were to transfer myself out of my chair and to roll over, both by myself. These are two very daunting tasks for a quadriplegic with little core and upper body strength. The staff at Kennedy Krieger didn't say, "No, you can't do that. That's not possible." They agreed. Each day at 9 a.m., I'd practice transferring out of a chair over and over until I was exhausted. Then I'd work on rolling over.

At noon, Mom would meet me for lunch. The days were tough on her because there really wasn't anywhere to go. That year was a difficult snowy winter, so by the time she got back to the hotel, she'd have to turn around and come back to Kennedy Krieger. Instead, she'd sit in the waiting area and read a book, do some research on rehabilitation facilities, or make phone calls. She waited so many hours for me, endless hours I can't even begin to count. And she never once complained or felt sorry for herself for missing out on the life she was supposed to be living. She and my dad had hoped that by this time in their life, after twenty-five years of marriage, they'd be free to travel and spend time together. Her commitment to me and my rehabilitation was a tremendous sacrifice, one for which I am forever grateful.

After lunch, I'd go to the gym on my own to use a hand bike or wrist weights. I suppose I could have just hung around until the afternoon session, but I was at Kennedy Krieger to gain as much strength as possible. Occupational therapy started at 2 p.m. and included dressing myself, practicing how to use the bathroom, using eating utensils—skills I learned when I was four and most people take for granted, but ones I needed to learn all over again. I had disliked this part at other facilities, but Kennedy Krieger made it fun. The truth is, I need to be able to dress myself and go to the bathroom by myself if I want to be independent again.

Afterwards, I had pool therapy twice a week. I *loved* pool therapy. Once a swimmer, always a swimmer. I am reminded that, yes, I will be able to swim again. Swimming competitively was tough, but it was exhilarating to be in the water. As I propelled myself forward, stroke after stroke, it was as if I was part of the water itself. My heart would pump, and I would push myself harder and harder until I touched the wall, finished my race, and looked at the clock for my time. There is something undeniable about being in the water, and now, during pool therapy, I felt exhilarated again—free, light, happy, and able to move.

The pool at Kennedy Krieger has a moveable floor, allowing me to stand. The floor would rise, bringing my body upright, and the next thing I knew, I would be standing 6 feet 4 inches tall, towering over the pool therapist, who would inevitably make a comment about my height. The buoyancy of the water allows a person to do so much more than they can do on land, with the goal of becoming stronger. This is another step closer to my goal of walking again.

Being back at home in Connecticut is always comforting, bringing a sense of normalcy. I was truly exhausted from my three weeks at Kennedy Krieger and needed the break. However, there are so many things I can't do at home due to lack of equipment, but I work hard with what I do have. After an eighteen-month wait time, my dad's company, Enzo Biochem, was able to purchase a Functional Electrical System (FES) so that I could continue my therapy on the bike at home. The FES costs about $20,000, which would have been impossible for us to purchase on our own and would never be covered by insurance. The FES works by stimulating selected muscle groups; for me it was my glutes, quads, and hamstrings. As technology has advanced, I have been able to stimulate other muscle groups as well.

The first few times setting me up on the FES took my mom over an hour as the stimulation pads have to be in precise spots on my body. The machine gives me enough stimulation to reach and maintain a given speed at a specific resistance. Not all quadriplegics who use the FES can feel their muscles contracting, but I can! Watching my muscles contract is very gratifying. My muscles are getting stronger, and I have worked up to an hour on the machine before my muscles are too tired to maintain the resistance. Whenever I use the FES, I am so thankful for my dad's company and their generosity. It's people like them who are helping me continue on my road to recovery.

On Monday, Wednesday, and Friday my mom and I are out the door to Gaylord in Wallingford by 8:30 a.m. We arrive around 9:15 so that I can change and be in the pool by 9:30 for a forty-five-minute physical therapy session. After pool therapy, I change back into dry clothes then go upstairs for physical therapy with the focus on transferring to and from my chair, which means working on core and upper body strengthening for about forty-five minutes.

When I first started working with Erika, leaning side to side was impossible. I would be sitting upright on a full-sized mat, which was raised onto a table with my legs hanging over the side and my feet on the floor. The objective was to lean to the right and push myself back up with my elbow and repeat this on the other side. Easy, right? For most, but for me it was impossible at first. Erika stacked mats on my sides so I didn't have to lean as far to the right or left. With practice and more practice, over about six months' time, I was able to eliminate the pads and lean all the way down to the mat, push myself up with my elbow, and repeat ten reps on both sides.

Another challenging exercise is sitting with several pads on my lap and leaning forward to put my chin on the pads. It requires tightening the back of my shoulder blades and neck and the strength in my core to lift myself up. After fifteen reps, Erika removes one pad and I repeat the exercise, then she removes the last pad so that I have to lean all the way down to my knees. Again, it may sound simple, but these basic tasks take a lot of energy for me to complete.

Next Erika helps to roll me over onto my stomach, which sometimes makes my legs very angry. They shake and spasm with the change in position frightening onlookers, but I don't mind the spasms. I actually love feeling the muscles in my legs move. Once my legs calm down and I'm lying flat on my stomach, Erika puts an inclined pad under my chest and helps me put skateboard-like roller scooters under my arms. She straps my arms on, and I roll them forward to straighten my arms and back so that my elbows reach my waist, while keeping my head up. Erika directs the scooter so it doesn't topple over, but my rhomboids and shoulder blades are doing the work. Continuing on my stomach with the inclined mat, I pull my arms back, pointing my elbows to the ceiling and pinching my shoulder blades together, then repeat. After my accident my shoulder blades were "kissing," so to speak. With therapy the muscles underneath my shoulder blades have become stronger and the blades don't touch any longer. This is huge progress for me and my steps toward being able to transfer in and out of my chair. As Erika says, "One day it will all come together."

We are home by 1 p.m. for lunch and then it's time to study. While I am in my standing frame doing classwork for online courses with Harvard, my mom finally gets a chance to shower and do a few things for herself. Being home allows us to do our own thing for part of the day. I like my space as much as she really needs her space. However, following a routine at home is equally as important as when I am at a rehabilitation center. It keeps me focused on getting stronger and working toward achieving my goals.

On June 14, 2015, I was accepted into the Harvard University Extension School to earn my degree in governmental studies—another step toward independence. It should take about two and a half years for me to complete the program and have a degree in government with a minor in psychology. I was able to get an extension for open-ended essay tests since my typing is limited to my left pinky. Based on when I graduated from high school, I should have graduated from college in May 2014. Most of my friends, like Kevin, have graduated and are working in "real" jobs now. When I see their lives moving ahead, it drives me to do the same. I could get jealous or frustrated, but instead I look ahead and picture myself doing something I love. Through this accident, helping people face challenges of their own has become a primary interest, along with understanding and supporting legal rights of those with disabilities like myself. I'm headed in the right direction, one step at a time.

CHAPTER 13

No Regrets

We cannot direct the wind, but we can adjust our sails.
—THOMAS S. MONSON[24]

At an inspirational talk I gave for a church youth group, an eighth grader asked, "Do you regret what happened to you? Are you angry at God for allowing you to become a quadriplegic?"

The question took me off-guard at first. It was the first time someone had the courage to ask me the question that looms over people who meet me and see a young guy with so much life ahead. I thought for a minute. The group was silent, waiting for my answer, when I said without a doubt in my voice, "No, I don't regret what happened to me." I explained my frustration at not being able to do whatever I want, whenever I want. So, do I wish my life were back to normal? Yes, but I have no regrets for the last six years of my life. God only gives a person as much as they can handle, making one a stronger person with each challenge faced.

"Have you experienced Post Traumatic Stress Disorder?" another girl asked. I learned later that she had been in a horrific car accident that changed her ability to cope. She became fearful of driving, and it halted her independence. PTSD was not a diagnosis for me. There were times when I felt down, but I was able to shake it off. Whether it was my family support, my attitude, or my faith, I don't know. I saw her shoulders slump and realized she wanted to hear that she was going to be okay, that her experience with PTSD was acknowledgeable, so I said, "While I wasn't diagnosed with PTSD, I dealt with depression and fears just like someone with PTSD. It's all part of the process." I don't know, but I hope my words helped her let go of the fear in order to move on. She had to give it up to God and know that He is guiding her along the way.

Talking to the group, I explained that I've learned to look ahead with my life plans and goals. There's no reason to look back and ask what ifs and whys. Six years ago, I didn't really have a life plan, living day by day, not really thinking about the future. When the accident happened, I had to grow up faster and think differently about myself and my life. Ironically, I have experienced a lot of things that I might otherwise have missed. I finished freshman year at the College of Charleston, and now I'm studying government and psychology at the Harvard Extension School and working part-time at Access Independence.

The people I have met would not have crossed my path if it hadn't been for my accident. My college swim teammates and I, nicknamed "The Goon Squad," were partiers. We often stayed out drinking late into the night and even into the morning, which made practices difficult at times, but that didn't stop us. Academics were not a priority at all, and I had no career direction in mind. Perhaps the accident was God's way of slowing me down before something worse happened. Sometimes I wonder if God actually saved me from myself. Maybe I wouldn't even be here if it weren't for the accident. I don't know for sure, but I often wonder. My belief is that God has a plan, a plan for me and for you.

After a talk I gave to a college gymnastics team, many of the gymnasts said they get caught up in the little stuff and take for granted the important things like being a healthy college athlete and student. I remember those days when studying and then going to practice every day was overwhelming and sometimes unbearable. Thinking back on that now, I realize my life was easier then, despite it feeling like nothing could be harder at the time. Another athlete said she was struggling with an injury that was preventing her from doing her sport and that things weren't going her way. After my speech, she realized that her injury was just a "bump in the road" and that once she had surgery, she'd be able to compete again, whereas someone in my shoes can never do that. Surgery is not a fix for a quadriplegic.

I reminded the athletes to hang with the friends who would understand and support them and provide strength like I did at the College of Charleston and do now. Most of my close friends from high school have been around for me. Ironically, they also come to me when they need someone to talk to, to help them sort through issues of their own. I've always listened and given my friends honest advice. A few friends did not come around once I was injured. For whatever reason, they couldn't handle seeing me in a bed with a halo attached to my head, or in a wheelchair, unable to walk. It's a loss when you have a friend from the time you were a toddler, one you were inseparable from, and then life changes and so does the friendship.

On the other hand, some people who were just acquaintances have gone out of their way to help, whether it was a donation, bringing food over, sending inspirational videos, helping transport me, building ramps for the house, or just a simple visit. A few friends stepped out of my life temporarily but have come back around and are apologetic about not seeing me through the worst. My response to them is that I don't hold any grudges. Everyone deals with conflict in different ways, but I'm always glad to have a friend back in my life.

Since I can't do the same things I used to do with my friends, get-togethers are different and sometimes even a bit stressful. There's not much to do at my house when friends come over. I want to just get up and go, but I can't do that on my own. My buddy Kevin will come over, help me into my mom's car—which we jokingly call "My Chariot" with the wheelchair access—and we'll go out to a bar, to the movies, or to another friend's house. He and I have taken up the hobby of IPA tasting together. Every so often we'll head over to Two Roads Brewing Company in Stratford, Connecticut, for a few beers and to just hang out and relax.

I told my audience of athletes about my first job as a quadriplegic working for Access Independence. The company, previously called Disability Resource Center of Fairfield County, provides support and jobs to people like me who have been injured and can't perform daily tasks independently. Their goal is to promote independence, educate, and provide services for the disabled. I get to help people like myself through the challenges of understanding benefits, finding equipment, and learning how to manage in a safe home.

On the first day, my mom and I arrived at Access Independence and ironically couldn't locate the handicap entrance. We had a good laugh since it was so ridiculous a situation. I spent the first few days at the job reading about the company and its procedures. The reading was partially about dealing with someone in a wheelchair. Ironic, huh? Much of the information I knew from my personal experience as a person in a wheelchair. For example, tip number one: if you are a walking person, don't ever pat the head of a person in a wheelchair. Sounds simple enough, but people actually do that, pat quads on the head. It's happened to me and it's a bit humiliating. Tip number two:

talk directly to the injured person, not the caretaker. As a disabled person, I can relate to this. Whenever I meet with a new provider or go to a new facility, the natural inclination for the doctor or whomever is to talk directly to my mom, not to me. She is great about it and always redirects them to ask me what *I* think.

Access Independence is a nonprofit federally funded organization that serves as a middleman to people with disabilities who are having difficulty getting the proper care or have questions about how to get the care. I answer the phone and direct the calls to the right person. I also sit in on initial meetings with clients, whether it's to help them get in-home care, find long-term housing, get an extension on a lease, procure equipment, or other reasons. The state has a deal with Access Independence, so my work there is like an internship. Initially, they paid for me to work up to 120 hours at $10 per hour. They ordered a Mac for me to work on and would even hire an aide to assist me with bathroom use, eating lunch, and anything I can't do by myself. The Bureau of Rehabilitation Services provides these services, because their goal is to get people with injuries back in the workforce and off Social Security. After six months, Access Independence had an opening for an Independent Living Advocate, and I was hired as an employee, no longer under the BRS.

At first I was working only four hours at a time and was always asking my boss for more work. I wanted this to be a real working experience. To work any longer than four hours would mean I might need to use the bathroom, which I can't do on my own *yet*, but hope to with time and practice. My brain does receive a signal that I need to pee; however, my hands are not fully functioning, so my mom or another caregiver inserts the catheter for me for now. I am also reliant on a caregiver for bowel movements—a process that takes about an hour and involves lying on a pad with a suppository placed into my rectum, usually by my mom. It's one thing when I am in the comforts of home, but another when out and about and food poisoning comes on quickly. There is no stopping the diarrhea. There's no getting to a bathroom quickly. It is one ugly mess that is upsetting, and for some, humiliating, but not for me. It is what it is.

One night I was out to eat with my mom and dad, and the food didn't sit well with me. By the time we pulled into the driveway, my parents had to carry me, run into the house, throw me down on a pad—and it was a mess. My mom yelled out, "Holy crap, Chris!" which set us all to laughing hysterically. You have to turn it around and laugh about it or it will drag you down. People have asked me if given the choice, would I rather have my bladder and bowel function back or be able to walk again. Unlike most paraplegics, as a quad I can honestly say that I would much rather walk again. There are always alternatives to using the bathroom, even if accidents happen.

I had been on a state waiting list since March 2014 to be trained to hire a caregiver. This had to happen for me to work more hours. The caregiver would come around noon, catheter me, help me eat lunch, and help me move around a bit. The purpose of having a job right now is to build confidence and experiences away from home and with a caregiver other than my mom. The reality is that my mom might not always be able to provide the same support as she is giving me now. It took until October 2015 to get the caregivers put in place. Eventually, we hired several caregivers, but for many reasons we have since gone back to our old routine.

It was never easy for me to sit still. Up until my accident, I was always on the go. I'd come home after high school or work and be out the door again to swim, sail, go to the fire department, or hang with friends. There was always something to do. Now, when work is slow, I wheel around the office to see what everyone else is doing, ask for more work, or roll up and down the hallway just to keep moving. Being bored and unable to get up and go is very challenging and annoying actually. Often, I flap my arms by my side and move them around in circles to keep circulation going while I'm sitting waiting. I spend a lot of time waiting for others to help me, which has made me a more patient person.

As a teen, I was egocentric and confident and took independence for granted. I was infallible, just like young athletes I have spoken to. My focus was on having adventures, being with friends, and spending as little time at home as possible. It never crossed my mind that life could change on a dime. As I speak to young athletes, I tell them that life won't always go according to their plan. There are no guarantees. There will be curve balls, there will be wins, and there will be losses. I tell them they need to keep faith, have a positive attitude, and harbor no regrets through those times.

CHAPTER 14

Change

God grant me the serenity to accept the things I cannot change,
the courage to change the things I can,
and the wisdom to know the difference.
—REINHOLD NIEBUHR[25]

C hange and facing the unknown is challenging for anyone. Change can also be positive if a person opens their mind and gets past the fear; they can meet new opportunities with optimism and be more successful in the end. I like to look at the changes in my life that way. At the beginning of the summer after my freshman year in college, I was independent, living my life day by day, sometimes on the edge, always thinking nothing could happen to me. Now my life, and that of my family, has changed in unimaginable ways over the past six years. Even so, I am the same person deep inside that I was before. I'm just sitting now instead of standing. My wheelchair doesn't define me. I don't want people to see me as a "quad"; I want them to see me as the same old fun-loving, optimistic, friendly Chris

O'Brien. So I was taken off-guard recently when a man at a rehab center said to me nonchalantly one day, "So you are a cripple too?"

I looked at him, shocked by his comment, and responded, "No, I have a handicap, I'm not crippled." The man shrugged his shoulders, not seeing the whole picture, not seeing beyond my wheelchair. Unfortunately, people who didn't know me before my accident can't always see beyond the wheelchair at first. There's a certain look. A look people give me of sorrow that I don't need or want.

Coming home after the accident and never going upstairs or downstairs in the house I lived in for seventeen years of my life was a difficult change. A task that was so simple and taken for granted was now impossible. The room I had made my own with first-, second-, third-place swim ribbons and trophies lining the shelves, pictures and posters adorning the walls, and other memorabilia was upstairs. Upstairs was now an unreachable place where all my belongings lived in an otherwise empty room. My bedroom is now in the old dining room off the kitchen, adjacent to the front door, bathroom around the corner, with an FES bike, a standing frame, a motorized bed, bureau, and a full-sized wall poster from a fundraiser that reads, "Music in the Grass...Helping Chris Walk Again." It's easily accessible in case of a fire so someone could get me out of the house quickly by wrapping me in a sheet and dragging me out the front door—not something that could be done from upstairs.

Previously, I'd also hang out in our "man cave" downstairs with family and friends playing Xbox and other games, watching sporting events and Netflix, and just relaxing. Those memories can't be forgotten when I'm surrounded by them above and below me every day. So when my parents said they were thinking about selling the house, my first feeling was sadness. Then I thought about it for a while and decided to look at it as a positive. This house is filled with old memories of growing up, twenty-plus years' worth now. I want to hold those memories in my heart, but perhaps it's time to make new ones as a family in a new place. After all, our life is different now than it was.

When it does happen, selling the house will ease some of the financial strain, but also allow us to be more flexible. At some point, I will need to be in Boston to attend a semester at Harvard to complete my degree. And we are always looking for rehabilitation places elsewhere that support my needs. Without the responsibility of owning a house, it will be more manageable for my parents. How that works for Matt, I'm not sure yet. Perhaps it will be easier for him to establish himself in a new location now that he's graduated from college.

The changes in my life have obviously had a huge impact on my family. My mom had to quit a lucrative job to become my permanent caregiver. My dad spent more time on his own, taking an apartment in Long Island for midweek when Mom and I went to rehab in another state for weeks and months on end. Ironically, Matt, who was more dependent on Mom growing up, came home from high school and college breaks to an empty house and had to fend for himself.

It's not all negative though. Despite being apart, our family has become closer on many levels. When life takes an unexpected turn for the worse, often families fall apart at the seams. In our case, the family bond grew deeper. Despite having to divide and conquer, my family is strong and has stuck together every step of the way. Mom would spend more time with me and Dad would spend more time with Matt. He would travel on fall weekends to Matt's soccer games, and they'd have dinner out together somewhere when they were both home. Matt and Dad are a lot alike; they both love to eat and neither is much of a talker, unlike Mom and me, who both need to talk things out and be on the go most of the time. So, while we were apart for periods of time, my brother and I both had a parent to rely on, and we kept in touch on a daily basis no matter the location.

Even relatives we hadn't spent much time with came around, and our relationships are stronger than before. Not only have my aunts and uncles, cousins and grandparents all been around for us, but we've had to be there for them too.

I see my friends going through big, but normal changes in their lives: graduating from college, getting jobs, moving to different areas, and leaving the hometown they grew up in. Leaving me behind at times too. Am I envious? Yes, but my goal of becoming independent outweighs that envy, because I truly believe God has a plan for me. Despite my life not going how I thought it might, I see a promising future down the road. When I first went to Shepherd Center a year after being injured, I remember telling Kevin that I'd be walking when I got home for Thanksgiving. That was not the case then and not the case now, but that can change if I stay optimistic and keep working at it. I'm reminded of Erika, one of my physical therapists, saying, "Chris, keep working at it and one day it will all come together." I have to believe that is the truth.

PART II

A ROSE, AN ANCHOR, AND A COMPASS

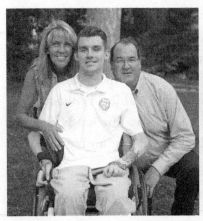

Chris with his Mom and Dad

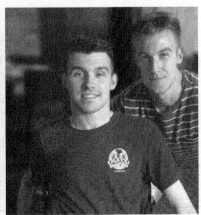

Chris and his brother, Matt

Once Mom got over her reaction to my first tattoo, she agreed to take me for a second. It reads "DETERMINATION," which has become my motto. In today's world, getting a tattoo helps people define who they are and what is important. With my additional tattoo, I thought about my family and the different roles each plays in my life. So my most recent tattoo, a rose, is for my mom. Some believe the white rose symbolizes Mary and her immaculate conception, representing the purity and holiness of Mary. There are many images of Mary, but the one titled Our Lady of Reconciliation depicts a heart crowned with white roses being pierced by a sword. To me, this represents that when a mother gives birth, she loves her children unconditionally, and she allows herself to be vulnerable. One of Mary's hands is pointing at her heart while the other is pointing outward, showing that a mother gives herself completely and shares the burdens and suffering of her children.

Other rose colors represent passion and sacrifice, wisdom and joy, gratitude and peace, wonder, awe, and change for the better. My mom bears the burden of my life daily. She makes sacrifices on my behalf daily and provides me with much wisdom and joy. Without her, I would not be in the positive place I am today. She is a bouquet of roses. The tattoos to follow would be an anchor for my brother and a compass for my dad.

Chapter 15

Carrie

For it is in giving that we receive.
—FRANCIS OF ASSISI[26]

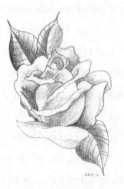

Unconditional Love

Chris and I have always been a team, going back to when he was a little kid through his elementary, middle, and high school years. Chris spent endless hours with me volunteering. He was always by my side whether it was at a food or clothing drive for the neighborhood improvement association, or when I was coaching Matt's St. Catherine of Siena Church basketball team. Chris was always willing to jump in, even as a five-year-old, and help without direction. Volunteering and helping others came naturally to both of us.

We also spent many hours traveling and supporting Matt at his soccer games. Matt played soccer from kindergarten through college, so we spent many afternoons and weekends, rain or shine, cheering Matt on from the bleachers. Chris was never really the athletic type, except for swimming, but he came to as many games as possible. That's what we do as a family; we support each other no matter what it takes. It's no wonder Matt has been there for Chris every step of the way as well.

Matt went off to college when Chris was in the throes of therapy. He would come home for holidays, summer break, and no one would be home. He'd stay with Lori and Jim, his aunt and uncle, or sometimes with friends. Otherwise he'd be coming home to an empty, quiet, cold house that used to be filled with laughter and warmth. A few times Matt came home with some friends from college and stayed at the house, and although he never complained, *I know* the loneliness that penetrated the walls of our formerly lively home was not the best for him. He missed what used to be, what might never be again. My life was focused on getting Chris the best therapy possible, even if it meant spending less time with Matt. My heart broke and I felt guilty when I imagined Matt home alone. Guilt is like bricks on my shoulders, hard to lift, but I always remind myself that I'd do the same for Matt.

Guilt carried over into my marriage. I couldn't focus on Paul anymore. The strongest of marriages would be strained under our circumstances. Between the financial stresses, traveling to different rehabilitation centers, getting Chris the right therapy, his daily care, and the fact that our boy was now a quadriplegic brought turmoil to our marriage of twenty-seven years. Our future, as we had imagined it, was on hold. Paul and I were close to having an empty nest. We had talked about relocating once the kids were in college and more independent. We imagined moving down South, perhaps near my mom and stepdad, where the boys could come for holidays and vacations. We imagined daily walks on the beach, golfing in the afternoons, and simply spending time together, just the two of us after all these years of parenting.

Now our talk was different. We put all our dreams for retirement aside when Chris had his accident. Now we sensed each other's worries about where to go from here, about our son's future, about our financial situation. Despite not always being on the same page in our thinking, we have a solid relationship that has been built on trust, values, and sticking together through the good and the bad, for better or worse.

Before the accident, I took an exciting but very demanding job with Macy's creating displays for holidays like Christmas. From there, my next position was on the sign team for the sales department. After that, I became a manager with the jewelry department just as the jewelry business exploded. I was working sixty-plus hours a week so I wasn't home very much. Paul traveled some, Matt and Chris were fending for themselves quite a bit, but they were so busy that it didn't appear to bother them. We were all happily going about doing our own thing, but coming together at night for dinner when possible.

Come springtime, I was getting burned out from the constant overtime. In May and June, the jewelry business was still booming, and I was working hard to hire and train the right people and keep sales up. It was very stressful trying to keep up with the numbers from September to April. Then, in an instant, everything changed when Chris dove innocently into Block Island Sound. There was no way around it. I had to leave a career that I had built for myself, just like that. My job would now be to take care of him on a full-time basis.

Strangely, when I went to clean out my office, a sense of relief washed over me, and I wondered if this was now God's plan for *me*. Whether I realized it or not at the time, I was ready for a change in my life—not of this magnitude, of course, but the timing was right for me to take a break from work. Macy's had been all-consuming and took me away from family life. Putting less than 110 percent into everything I do is not an option for me. I tend to jump overboard, but that is my personality. On the other hand, being thrown into a tragic, life-altering situation was daunting. Suddenly I was bound to home and to Chris. No more leaving to walk with friends, or do errands, or just go to the gym. My life would not be my own anymore, perhaps indefinitely. I went from a career in retail working sixty hours a week to being a caregiver 24/7. Just like Chris, though, I never asked "Why me?" or "Why Chris?" It is what it is.

For now, I have to think in chunks of time. I can't plan where Paul and I, Matt, or Chris will be ten years from now; it's just not manageable. Right now, it's a matter of getting Chris as strong as possible and able to live independently. Many amazing people have come into my life because of Chris's accident. Many have left my life too. I've grieved over the loss of some friends, good friends who could not handle my new life circumstances. I've learned, too, that some people have different philosophies than Paul and I do. Some parents actually abandon their children who are paralyzed with spinal injuries. They basically leave them in bed to die or in the hands of others who don't help them get stronger, who don't believe in them, who don't push them to walk again.

It boggles my mind that a mom could leave her child, her baby, but some do. Some have even suggested that Chris's brother, Matt, should be his primary caregiver, that he should give up his life goals to assume the responsibility now that he's graduated from college. When I gave birth to my boys, it was forever. I will do whatever it takes to support them, to encourage them to achieve and pursue their lifetime dreams, whatever they may be. They have always come first in my life, so now my life is about helping Chris walk again.

Friends know me as a planner, and I was usually the organizer of neighborhood family events: annual football tailgates at the Harvard vs. Yale football game, tubing down the Farmington River, barbeques at the lake. These planning and organizational skills have been extremely useful over the past six years. Everything we do now has to be strategically thought out. Just going out to dinner as a family needs to be arranged in advance. We need to make reservations including room for a wheelchair. Otherwise we could arrive and not be able to get Chris to the table.

One time we went to a restaurant and the hostess had to lead us through the kitchen to get to our table. Another time we went to a Travelers PGA Tournament which unbelievably did not have handicap access. We had to bring Chris in his chair through a tent that was wet, grassy, and difficult to maneuver. Security wouldn't let Chris go on the cart path, so he pushed himself through the muck without a grumble. Later, Chris wrote a letter to Travelers on his work letterhead, Access Independence, explaining what had happened with the hopes of making it better for the next handicapped person with tickets to a PGA tournament. He never received a response.

Whenever we go to a new building, a store, a mall, anywhere, we have to leave time to find the handicap entrance. Surprisingly, access to buildings is not made simple for handicapped people. We've learned that the hard way driving around buildings, looking for ways to get Chris inside.

There is so much we still don't know about how to get Chris back on his feet again. One thing we *do* know is that we can never give up or give in to the challenges that lie ahead. We have to be his advocate. No single directory or book provides a step-by-step action plan on how to take care of our son. We've had support from rehabilitation centers, but we've had to figure out the majority on our own. Way back in the beginning, while we were at Shepherd in Atlanta, Chris was told that I needed to go through training on how to catheterize him. I'd already been doing that for three months, and I was pretty darn sure I was doing it right. Chris hadn't had any infections or problems. Yet still I had to join in the training. Some things we just had to do.

Faith and hope keep me going every day. I attend mass at times, and on many occasions the Gospel or the readings speak to me. On Good Shepherd Sunday, the Gospel reading was from John 10:18, which reads, "No one takes my life from me, but I have power to lay it down and power to take it up again. This command I have received from my Father." After the reading, Father Marcello spoke of a man who had lost his arm in WWII. A surgeon had to amputate and wanted to tell his patient himself. When the man woke up from surgery, the surgeon said, "I'm so sorry, but you've lost your arm." The man replied, "I did not lose my arm, I gave my arm for France."

Of course, Chris came to mind. Chris has chosen not to feel sorry for himself, but to see the good in the path God has chosen for him. We don't always see God's plan clearly in front of us. It can take years to understand, even a lifetime. While Chris does not see it, his faith and determination have touched many lives, providing a positive influence for others since his accident—the numbers are infinite.

I believe it's all part of the plan. This would not have happened if Chris wasn't a strong person to teach others through his story. You also don't survive this kind of accident without faith, without someone watching over you. I feel God's presence guiding us and watching over us all the time. It may sound silly, but every time we go somewhere, there's a parking spot right outside. Every time we go somewhere, there is a person who helps us. Every time we go somewhere, we learn something new about this journey.

It took me over a year to be able to talk to other people about Chris's accident. I don't remember people reaching out to me for help until we were at Shepherd. At Shepherd, people sought us out. They wanted *our* input and thoughts on next steps when we weren't experts ourselves. We were there for an extended stay, so our name became known. One family in particular, whose son Shaun was paralyzed from the waist down in a car accident, said to me one day, "How does Chris do it? How does he stay positive and happy mentally and work so hard physically toward recovering and walking again?"

Chris has made an impression on other people from earlier in his life and the new ones he's met during this journey, despite his not seeing it that way. Chris has friends who still call him for advice with issues, problems, and girls. They look up to him because he is someone they can trust. Chris is a straight-honest-truth kind of person that people gravitate toward.

Several years ago, a boy named Tucker who lived in Virginia had a similar accident to Chris's while at a beach in Delaware. He also dove into a wave and was instantly paralyzed. While Chris did not know Tucker, nor Tucker know Chris, they were brought together at Shepherd in Atlanta. Meg's sister, Deb, whom I had met and spent time with, knew Tucker's mom, Roxanne. As it turned out, Tucker would be starting therapy at Shepherd while Chris and I were there. Meg gave me Roxanne's phone number. We chatted a few times, but it wasn't until another visit to Shepherd that Chris and Tucker became friends, and Roxanne and I began spending time together.

In the beginning, the grief is so great for a quadriplegic and his family that it's difficult to reach out or open up to new people, even if they are trying to help. Over time, we became very good friends and have helped each other in ways that I believe were also part of the plan. A world of people we would never have met have crossed our paths because of Chris. I cherish these new friendships.

CHAPTER 16

Matt

―――

Anchor: A person or a thing that provides support or strength.[27]

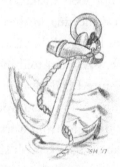

Support and Strength

Chris and I have always been close. Being only two years apart, we were constantly together in our toddler and elementary days. In middle school and high school, though, we went our separate ways. Chris was never home; he was off swimming or sailing, day in and day out. I was on the high school soccer team, hanging out with friends, and very busy myself. Even though our lives had gone different ways, we were still brothers, brothers who would do anything for each other.

When I got the call from Kevin that Chris had been in an accident, that he had hit his head, I figured at first they had been cliff jumping at the Housatonic River, one of Chris's favorite things to do. He spent many summer days with friends at the river where there was a rope swing and cliffs to jump from. Our parents always warned Chris to be careful, so he'd tell Mom and Dad that he'd scoped out the water and was sure there were no rocks or dangers in his way. He was the risk taker, the "Wild Child" we called him.

On the other end of the phone, Kevin's voice sounded shaky: "Matt, there's been an acc...acci...accident." For Kevin to be so upset, I knew the situation was not good. I called my mom, who was on her way home from a business meeting in the Hartford area, about an hour away. That was when I learned that Chris was actually in Block Island, not close to home. My mom told me to go to Fairfield and stay with my Aunt Barb since I had to work early the next morning teaching a soccer clinic. She and my dad would be going straight to Rhode Island once they got home from work. Not wanting to worry me, my parents didn't elaborate on Chris's situation when we spoke that night, though her voice was different. It was flat, businesslike, holding back the truth. I knew.

On Saturday, two days after the accident, my mom came back from Rhode Island to pick me up and return to Rhode Island Hospital. She warned me that Chris was in bad shape and that I should prepare myself for seeing him in the halo brace. I tried to visualize Chris as my mom described him, but nothing could prepare me for what I would see. Finally, we arrived at Rhode Island Hospital. I loathe hospitals: the smells, the noises, the quiet, the doors you have to enter to get from one place to another. I imagine getting lost in a hospital and not being able to find my way out. It's like a bad dream. That's how much I hate hospitals.

We went inside, gave our names at the front desk, and were handed visitor badges for the ICU. We took the elevator to the sixth floor. With the loud ding, I remember stepping off the elevator and feeling a large pit in my stomach. I walked slowly down the hallway noticing people in full comas, monitors beeping everywhere, families holding hands, crying, sadness... Then the hall was bright, and as I turned the corner to enter Chris's room, I burst into tears. He was just lying there with this contraption bolted to his head. Heavily sedated, his body was swollen and puffy, and he couldn't speak. He couldn't move any part of his body except his dark-brown eyes, which focused on the ceiling and rolled ever so slowly to the right to look at me. Our eyes met, and I saw him telling me, "Don't worry, bro. I've got this. I'll be fine. We're good."

Chris has always been the most positive, strong-willed, and determined person I've ever known, next to my mom, that is, even as a child. I was holding my breath and had to tell myself to relax, but I didn't really know what to do, what to say, how to act. I couldn't just sit there, so I reluctantly put my hand on his shoulder and made small talk. I talked, babbled about this, that, and the other thing without asking any questions since he couldn't answer. When we left the hospital that day, I couldn't stop the picture in my mind of Chris lying there motionless. What would he do? How could he stay like that? Driving back home, I hid my tears under my sunglasses. Mom and I both cried the whole way home. No words could make things better.

Word started to get around town about Chris. People asked a lot of questions. Everywhere I went, someone would ask me, with empathy, how Chris was doing, how were my parents coping, and how was *I* doing? It was as if Chris were dead. I seriously thought that Chris would be walking within a few months, so I'd say he was coming home soon and that he was going to be fine. Well, Chris did not come home as soon as I had thought he would, and he wasn't walking in a few months either. The seriousness was beginning to sink in, and my life was suddenly very different without my big brother at home.

In August 2011, my senior year in high school began with my mom and dad back and forth to Gaylord Rehabilitation Center in Wallingford where Chris was moved once released from the hospital. School, college applications, and soccer kept me very busy and distracted from Chris at times. The seriousness of the matter finally sank in when, one day over the morning announcements, the principal talked about Chris. He asked everyone to say prayers for Chris O'Brien and his family and for Chris to recover from this "tragic" accident.

Tragic. The word exploded in my head, the reality striking like a bolt of lightning. The room went silent; only the voice over the PA was heard. I put my head down on my desk, like no one was there, and sobbed. I sobbed uncontrollably listening to the announcement continue: "Bracelets will be sold in the cafeteria as a fundraiser for Chris O'Brien's rehabilitation." My teacher put a hand on my shoulder and asked if I needed anything. Did I need anything? Yes. I needed my brother back. I needed this tragedy to go away. As it turned out, my good friends Dan and Keith had come up with the idea of selling bracelets in support of Chris and wanted the school to be involved. They had two thousand blue bracelets made with the logo "CHRIS O'BRIEN...DETERMINATION." About $7,000 later, every single bracelet was sold. Everywhere I looked, people I didn't even know were wearing the bracelet for Chris's sake.

I had to grow up and become independent faster. I'd always been rather dependent on my mom, to say the least. She's just that kind of mom. She made me food, did my laundry, took care of me without a complaint. I think she actually loved it. When Chris had the accident, my mom wasn't home anymore; she was with Chris somewhere, wherever the therapy was that could be provided at the time. When I went off to college the following year, I'd come home for breaks and no one was there. Imagine coming home that first time. After years of coming home to a house full of people laughing and sharing stories, now it was eerily quiet, empty, and lonely.

I'd walk up the ramp with a pit in my stomach thinking about Chris, then into the side door where I was usually met with the smell of food being prepared and the sound of Mom either chatting on the phone, visiting with friends in the kitchen, or watching the news while she cooked dinner, then she'd holler, "Matt, you're home!" But now when I entered the house I could hear a pin drop, and smell the empty smell of an unlived-in house. It's such a strange feeling unlocking the door, walking in, dropping my bag on the floor, and hearing in my head, "Hey, bro. Welcome home." Instead, I would drop my bag and walk from room to room noticing how everything was left. It's funny what you notice—a paint chip here, an empty vase there that would have otherwise been filled with live flowers. Tears would fill my eyes as I picked up a family photo from the mantle, remembering the old times, the way things used to be before…before life changed…before Chris's accident.

I would try to fill the space by turning on the lights and the TV thinking that would help, but it didn't. Nothing can fill this empty space.

CHAPTER 17

Paul

Compass: To surround; encircle[28]

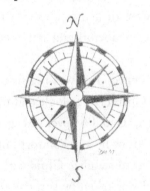

Pointing the Way

For whatever reason—I can't recall—I left work a bit early the day of Chris's accident. While driving home on I-95, I was entering traffic near Co-op City in the Bronx when I got Carrie's call.

"Chris is hurt. He can't move," she said hurriedly.

My first thought was, *He went to hang out at the beach. How could he be hurt?* The urgency in Carrie's voice nagged at me the rest of the drive home. I began praying and couldn't get home fast enough. When I arrived, Carrie was waiting for me, the car running, and she was anxious to get on the road to Chris in Rhode Island. We hit a lot of traffic, and being the impatient one, I took Siri's advice and got off the highway—only to encounter an even greater sea of brake lights. The traffic had us very uptight and arguing at first until we both fell silent, deep into our own worlds, for the remainder of the ride.

The sun set, and darkness crept into the sky and into our thoughts. After what seemed like forever, we arrived at Rhode Island Hospital around 9:30 p.m. and followed signs to the Emergency Room. Upon entering the ER, we were rushed to a room where Chris was being assessed by the emergency doctors and staff. The lights shone bright, but the mood was very serious and dim. Chris lay still on a gurney looking cold and frightened. This was the first and one of the only times I have ever seen Chris cry. He looked at me with worried, tear-filled eyes and muttered, "Dad, I'll never sail again." My heart sank at his words, and I didn't know how to comfort him.

The doctors decided to stabilize Chris with a halo brace. When they cut off his shirt, I was taken by surprise to see a very intricate tattoo of a Gaelic cross covering his shoulder.

"What the heck?" Carrie blurted out, but then Chris raised his arm slightly in my direction, which made me think he couldn't be paralyzed if he could raise his arm. This put my mind at ease for the moment. Carrie's reaction didn't surprise me, but everything was put into perspective when the medical team took Chris to the ICU.

It was late, and we were exhausted physically and emotionally. A nurse gave us some warm blankets so we could get some sleep in the lounge, which was dimly lit, empty, and quiet. My six-foot-six body didn't fit well on a hospital couch, so I was uncomfortable and unable to sleep for more than fifteen minutes at a time. It wasn't much better for Carrie. We had a few conversations between short stints of sleep, and even though Carrie and I were there together, the quiet of the room made me feel lonely and scared. This would be the beginning of many more sleepless nights for both of us.

The doctor came out of the ICU to see us at 4 a.m. He said the MRI showed a significant injury and bruising to the spine, and he mentioned levels C4-5. I remember thinking that the situation was bad, but it wasn't as bleak as it could be. I understood that Chris's spine was damaged but not completely severed, and he had a serious injury to level C4-5 that would require surgery. At that point, however, they just wanted to stabilize him. He was in no condition for a surgical procedure. So the plan was to keep Chris in the halo and monitor him every minute in the ICU.

The first couple of weeks were extremely challenging. It was difficult to leave the hospital, to come home not only without Chris, but also without Carrie. She stayed by Chris's side around the clock, even slept in the room, but I had to get home to Matt and back to work. My office was now in Long Island, a two-hour commute, and I was traveling a lot to England. One of the first days after the accident, Matt asked me if Chris was going to be all right, and I simply said, "I don't know, Matt. I really don't know."

Then Chris got pneumonia.

The doctors made it quite clear how dire this was for Chris's state of being. For the first time in my life, I thought Chris might die. Imagining life without him, without my son, took my breath away. Your child is not supposed to go before you. I didn't say this to Carrie or anyone else, nor did I let my tears be seen. Instead, I would spend time at the chapel and pray. I prayed for Chris's healing, for the strength to have the right words, to take care of my family, to take away my worries.

Overnight, our financial situation became daunting. Carrie had to stop working to be with Chris, and I had to work harder to keep our family afloat. My concerns were also for Chris and his future. Ironically, just one week before the accident, we had gone down to South Carolina to watch Matt play in a soccer tournament. While there, I signed a lease for an apartment and even bought a bed for Chris's fall semester at the College of Charleston. Come January, after paying tuition and rent for five months, we finally faced the truth and told the college that Chris would not be returning, ever.

Family support has been never ending. During Chris's rehabilitation at Shepherd in Atlanta, we spent weekends with Linda and David, Carrie's mom and stepdad. Chris was making progress and we all had high expectations, perhaps a bit unrealistic, but we were beginning to see some light. At times, the doctors and nurses didn't share our optimism, but that was not going to stop Chris from setting goals and determining to walk again.

Finally, Chris was accepted for rehabilitation at Kennedy Krieger, where our hopes became a reality. Kennedy Krieger asked Chris to set goals, and they would work to help him achieve them. Chris was, and still is, all business during his rehab there, and the staff is amazed at his progress each time he goes back for therapy. They love having him there because he is so motivated. When I see a therapist shed tears of joy while working with Chris, I know that every ounce of hard work on all our parts is worth it.

Not all parents can say they are inspired by their own kids, but Chris has taught me life lessons. I am admittedly a very impatient person, but Chris has made me a more patient person. He's taught me about having determination and discipline in my own life. I work hard, but Chris works even harder, every day. I have a positive attitude most of the time, but Chris has a positive attitude that never wavers. I smile, but Chris's smile lights up a room. We go out a lot, and people are taken off-guard by his smile, charisma, and personality because they shine.

I don't know if I could handle myself in Chris's situation with the same amount of patience, determination, discipline, and positivity. When I was eleven, I hit my head and saw stars. I think now, it could have happened to me. It could have happened to any of us. Chris wasn't doing anything stupid. He didn't get drunk and fall off a balcony. He simply dove into the water from the beach. The difference is, it takes a certain kind of person to handle such a situation and not give up on life.

When asked if I think Chris will walk again, my answer is absolutely yes. It may not be pretty, and it may not be perfect, but Chris *will* walk. Not only is he getting stronger every day, but his muscles are showing movement. That paired with technology? I know it will happen. Maybe not for some years, but it will happen.

Sometimes I think about where I see Chris in five years. After graduating from Harvard, I can see him going on to law school or working for the government where physical limitations are manageable. Most importantly, my hope for Chris is that he can have independence, a career, and a family someday. For right now, though, he needs us. He also needs a car. I want him to be able to say, "I'm going out," perhaps with a girl, or to work, or just to be with friends. Chris has filled all the requirements for getting a car, but we are waiting on the state. The red tape really tests my patience. Sometimes I just want to go out and buy him a car, but the cost is exorbitant.

Most likely Chris will always need our support in some way, but then don't most kids need their parents even as adults? At some point, we might need to move, perhaps closer to Kennedy Krieger, but for now we are all in a good place. In actuality, we've had more laughs than tears over the past six years as a family. The experiences we've had are not what we expected, but we make sure to have fun and take life one step at a time.

Chapter 18

Grandpa David and Nan

With determination, perseverance, and grit, there are no limits.

Grandpa David

Wednesday, July 27, 2011, was the day our family's lives all changed. An event that occurs tens of millions of times *every single day* around the world became a life-altering occurrence. Who could have predicted that something as common as diving into the surf during a summer idyll could touch so many lives?

The "butterfly effect" comes to mind. It's a poetic notion that the flap of a butterfly's wings in Brazil can set off a torrent of currents in the atmosphere that, weeks later, generates the formation of a tornado in the US. Yet this is what happened to us. It is our story for the rest of our lives, and while it may not be the one we would have chosen, we have all learned to adjust and adapt to the hand we've been dealt. As a result, we are also all thriving, none more so than Chris.

What has impressed us most, I think, is the innate intelligence and intellectual curiosity that has become apparent within Chris as he wends his way through Harvard. Perhaps that bump on the head knocked some smarts loose! The mere fact that, after taking a couple of courses online at other institutions, he took it upon himself to look into Harvard, take two classes (which he aced), then apply and be accepted to its Extension School, has always amazed us. The initiative and willingness to gamble on a dream took real courage. The fact that he has done so well in his studies has left us darn near speechless and, more importantly, has taught him (and us) that he can do anything he puts his mind to. He'd be the first to admit that he did not exhibit a serious academic tendency during his time at Charleston.

Perhaps it is indeed true that when one door closes, another opens.

Nan

How do I put everything I might say about Chris into one short essay? My thoughts and emotions swirl every time I think about Chris and his accident. I try not to think about the latter, for it is too painful to recall. The former I think about every day with sadness over what happened and enormous pride in what Chris has become. So I thought I might best tell a different story about Chris, which captures in large part how he has handled the last six years.

In 2002, I was diagnosed with cancer of the bladder. I was very scared about what might become of me. Once the diagnosis was confirmed, I had an operation to literally scrape away the cancer from the walls of my bladder. After that, the doctors told me I might have to lose the bladder and wear a urostomy bag for the rest of my life. For those who know me, this was a terrible thing to contemplate. Then one day, while riding in a car with Carrie, Chris, and Matt, we were discussing the cancer and what might happen. Chris, at age ten, suddenly said, "Nan, you're not going to lose your bladder."

I asked him, "How do you know?"

He said simply, "I just know." From the mouths of babes—but it made me feel so much better.

A couple of weeks later, I was at Carrie's house talking about the situation with her, and I started to cry and asked, "Why me?!"

Without hesitation, Carrie said, "Why not you?" Then she continued, "This is just something we have to deal with." Who knew at the time how prophetic that would be?

Later, I remember trying to make a deal with God. I said, "I can do this, I'll be okay. Just don't let anything happen to my grandchildren." Today, I can only think about the irony of that moment. Chris was right, of course. I was lucky enough not to lose my bladder. But then to have the accident happen—it's almost more than I can bear. As I write this, I can't help but think of the song "Unanswered Prayers."

On the other hand, I look now at the last six years, and I see how Chris and the whole family have come through the other side, and I can't help but be extremely proud of them all. Chris will be fine and a Harvard graduate soon! I still can't think about that day six years ago and the weeks and months that followed—it's still too painful—but I can see now that, as Chris's Grandpa wrote, "When one door closes, another one opens."

CHAPTER 19

Aunt Lori

C hris marched to the beat of his own drum as a young kid and then as a teen. He was different from the other boys in the family. He enjoyed BMX while Matt and his cousins Jon and Rob played soccer and baseball. Chris was a divergent thinker, while the other boys followed the traditional path. Chris talked about going to a local private high school with a new group of people, while the others never questioned attending public school with all their friends. In the end, he went to Trumbull High School and had the same guidance counselor as all the other O'Brien kids. The counselor remarked, "There is something about Chris that stands out, something special. I can't put my finger on it, but Chris is going to do something great with his life." She wasn't the only one who recognized Chris's uniqueness.

A few weeks before the accident, not knowing it would be their last for a long time, Carrie and Paul went out of town for a short vacation. They asked me and Jim, my husband and Paul's brother, to keep an eye on Chris and the house. Carrie suspected Chris would have people over, which is exactly what he did. One evening, Jim took a drive by the house and noticed a bunch of cars in the driveway and parked on the street. He went around the back and looked in the window to see beer cans and bottles lined up on the table and a bunch of carefree teenagers having a good ol' time.

When Jim called from his car to tell me, I texted Chris and said, "Get your butt over here." He knew I meant business when he coolly walked in the door, cap on backwards as usual. I took his hat off his head and smacked him with it. "What in God's name were you thinking?" That was just weeks before the accident. Carrie and Paul grounded him for a month upon their return, but for whatever reason allowed him to go to Block Island a few weeks later. I think about the irony of all these things that lined up for Chris. Jim, in his joking kind of way, said to Chris later, "You're probably lucky this accident happened to you. Who knows where you'd be otherwise."

On the day of the accident, I was in New York City with Jon signing a lease for an apartment when Jim called and said Chris was in a water accident and was being airlifted to Rhode Island Hospital. In shock, I said, "I don't get it. What happened?"

"Chris dove into a sandbar. No one knows yet what it means."

I knew right then everything was different; life had just changed for all of us. The memories of the other two people in my life who broke their necks, one who committed suicide years later, and the other who died from the injury, haunted me while I drove back to Connecticut and then up to Providence. Ironically, they were both swimmers. Do swimmers think they are invincible in the water? Upon arriving at the hospital, Jim and I were greeted by Kevin and Pat with tears of anguish. I took Pat by his broad, athletic shoulders, looked into his worried eyes, and said, "You saved a life. This is horrible, but it could be much worse."

"I just feel so guilty," was his response. Later, Chris would sincerely tell his friends it wasn't anyone's fault. Even so, the impact of this accident on his friends was irreversible. It was life changing for all of us, and especially for them at such a young, vulnerable age.

When Chris was sent to Gaylord for rehabilitation, I tried to help as much as possible. Jon was there by Chris's side too. This was as much for Jon, with his own illness of epilepsy, as it was for Chris. The two boys became very close. From August to November, Matt lived with us. He and my daughter Katelyn, only nine months younger, became very close also as a result of their brothers' health. It was senior year in high school with college applications to be done and senior events that started from the beginning of the school year; Carrie was away with Chris, and Paul was traveling with work. The impact of Chris's accident went deep. Even so, Matt didn't miss a beat despite being worried and very thoughtful about his brother. Matt grew up a lot, in a positive way. He was forced to be independent and to stay focused on completing college applications, when he could have given up hope. In the face of adversity, Matt, Katelyn, Jon, and Chris have all shown incredible strength of character.

Unfortunately, during this time I neglected my own health and frequently dealt with fatigue and stomach issues that are not pretty to describe. One day I couldn't help transfer Chris from his bed to his chair. My strength was gone, pain engulfed my stomach, and I just couldn't lift him. At that moment, it hit me. Something was very wrong. Symptoms I had ignored because there wasn't time for myself now refused to be denied. When you travel by plane, the airline always says to put the oxygen mask on yourself first, then help the person next to you. I learned this simple lesson the hard way. In life, to take care of others, you also need to take care of yourself *first*.

Being diagnosed with stage 3 colon cancer was devastating. Like Chris, I felt sorry for myself for all of about five minutes. Between knowing Chris and Jon were kicking their own health issues, I had to do the same. After nearly losing my son Jon to a massive seizure, along with Chris's current state, surviving colon cancer was something I just had to do. A surgical procedure to remove the cancer, followed by chemotherapy with its physical and mental side effects, were just challenges that had to be met face to face. My nephew—to whom I had preached taking responsibility for your actions—taught me not to give in to my disease. I tell Chris all the time that he saved me.

In 2015, Jon had invasive brain surgery. A battery that was supposed to last five years was implanted in his brain. Responsive nerve sensors would intercept seizures. After only two years, the battery stopped working, so another surgery was performed. We almost lost Jon that day when he seized on the operating table. He went into cardiac arrest, so it was a miracle he survived.

I used to hate when people would say, "God only gives people what they can handle," but honestly it's true. Collectively, the O'Brien family is made up of survivors—people who support each other and remain hopeful, faithful, and determined to live life to its fullest despite facing huge challenges. Carrie said over drinks one night, "It's a privilege to see what these kids are made of." From the outside looking in, people see a family that has faced tremendous challenges. Sometimes they pity us. In reality, we aren't sitting around crying; instead we are laughing our socks off together, creating a new normal.

PART III

DETERMINATION

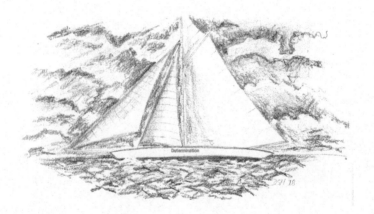

CHAPTER 20

Meg's View of Therapy

W hen I learned Chris would be at Kennedy Krieger Institute in Baltimore the same time I would be in Baltimore with my husband, who was attending a Firefighter's Convention, it gave me an opportunity to see him during rigorous physical therapy at one of the best SCI institutes in the country. I arrived at Kennedy Krieger with Carrie, who has had to master getting around Baltimore on her own with its one-way roads and trolleys bustling through intersections. Not only the driving can be challenging, but finding parking lots with handicap access, places to eat where Chris can enter the building not through a back door in the kitchen but through a main entrance, and finding handicap bathrooms outside of Kennedy Krieger where Chris, with the help of his mom, can use his catheter—all things most people take for granted are daily challenges for Chris and his mom, who spend every day together.

The first stop was the fourth floor where Chris was in PT. We sat in a cheerful white and purple lobby surrounded by other parents and caregivers waiting for their children, young men, and young women. On the wall in large script, a quote read, "In my mind, I am full of hope." Finding and having hope for recovery is the philosophy of Kennedy Krieger Institute. Sitting around waiting, listening, and observing, I was amazed by the lively environment. Moms, dads, and caregivers sat around chatting, listening to each other, sharing ideas for dealing with situations, and brainstorming how to deal with issues that come up. Every day offered a new situation to deal with whether it be insurance, scheduling procedures, or requesting services with no immediate solution.

At noon, the patients rolled out of the PT room one after the other to greet their parent or caregiver and head to level 2 for lunch at the café. Taking over several tables, we joined two other patients, JD and Will, and their moms for lunch. Chris, JD, and Will all met at Shepherd in Atlanta and have kept in touch, setting up therapy at Kennedy Krieger for the same weeks.

Looking around the lunch area, I saw a young girl about thirteen years old in a wheelchair. Her caregiver appeared to be an unhappy older sister. The patient was trying to get her sister to talk to her, but the sister rolled her eyes, shrugged her shoulders, told her to leave her alone, and continued texting on her phone. Unfortunately, this *does* happen, but not for Chris. Chris and Carrie go along their day in a routine and caring fashion.

After lunch, it was back up to the fourth floor for an hour of downtime before physical therapy began again. Everyone in the lobby appeared to be working: Carrie was updating FAFSA information for college loans they needed for Chris and Matt, Chris worked on homework for Harvard, Jackie was making phone calls to her insurance company, and JD and Will were both on their phones checking emails and messages. It was quiet, and I knew not to ask questions right then. Instead, I sat observing and taking in the normalcy of an abnormal situation.

At exactly 2 p.m., Ashley, Chris's PT, and her intern, Allie, came to get Chris while other PTs also entered the lobby and called for their patients. The lobby came to life as patients rolled themselves back into the PT room, surrounded by a wall of full-sized windows overlooking a walkway with gardens and the city. The place soon bustled with activity, each patient doing something different. Every patient had a different injury, disease, or complication to the spinal cord, each with a different level of functioning. Two people with the same injury can also have very different levels of functioning. In one area, a young man who had just graduated from college was using a Therastride™, where he was hoisted upright with braces around his legs and stimulation pads, allowing him to walk. Another physical therapist was pumping air into the tires of an arm bike that JD would use outside to roll around the courtyard. Will was practicing using a fork and spoon to pick up food. An older man was on the FES bike, and a young boy was using a walker to get around the room. Smiles, chatter, and laughter between the patients and their therapists filled the room, making it a very inviting place. All the while, high-fives and celebratory remarks encouraged each patient.

One of Chris's main goals at the time was to transfer in and out of his wheelchair by himself. So on this day the first activity was to get out of the chair onto a table cushioned with a mat similar to a double bed in size but level with the height of Chris's wheelchair seat. The mat was to his right, and the first step was to slide his rear end forward in his chair. Then the trial and error began. Allie attached padded handlebars onto each side of the chair, which Chris then wrapped his arms around at the elbow to try to lift himself up and shift toward the table. When that didn't work, Allie and Chris discussed what might work better, and she moved the handlebars around to the back of the chair facing outward so that Chris could wrap his left arm around the handlebar and shimmy himself to the right.

With his right arm, Chris had a rounded board with a Velcro strap and a loop to grab onto which allowed him to push the board slightly under his rear end—not an easy task without fully functioning arms and hands. After several attempts, once somewhat secured under his right butt cheek, Chris put his chest on his knees and moved his hips to the right, with help from Allie, onto the mat. This maneuver alone took about fifteen minutes, and Chris was not happy about needing some assistance. This surprised me as I have never seen Chris frustrated and annoyed before. He was quiet, serious, focused, and determined to complete the task independently.

While sitting on the matted table, Allie wrapped pads around Chris's arms to keep his elbows from buckling for the next exercise. She put stimulation pads on his back and triceps to stimulate contraction of the muscles and help him sit up straight. Then with his hands flat on the mat behind him, Chris walked his hands and bum backward and then forward again with the objective of strengthening his arms and shoulder muscles to help make transferring easier.

After repeating the exercise ten times or so, with the stimulation pads still on his back but taken off his triceps, Allie wrapped a 12-inch-wide band around his waist and around her waist, making a loop around the two of them. This allowed Chris to sit up taller. Lifting his arms to a 90-degree angle and down again was not too difficult, so Ashley added a target for Chris to touch and then lean toward to work the core. Chris repeated this exercise, with a few close falls, over and over until his muscles became too tired, at least a half hour.

Next came standing. Weight-bearing activities like standing are important for keeping bone density levels up in the legs. Chris's levels were at -4 whereas -2.5 is normal. Stimulation pads were placed on Chris's shoulders, lower back, butt, and thighs. The resistance was set based on his nerve and muscle sensation. For standing, a harness was wrapped around Chris's upper and lower body in case his leg muscles had spasms, which they often do. Using a harness, Chris was then lifted to a standing, upright position. His height of six-foot-four is quite surprising after seeing him sitting most of the time. "Oh my God, Chris. I didn't realize just how tall you are until now," remarked one of the therapists with a chuckle.

While Chris stood in the standing frame, another patient across the room on the Therastride™, along with several PTs, was playing Trivial Pursuit. They were struggling with some answers.

"What is the oldest city in the US?" we heard one ask.

Chris and I hollered in unison, "St. Augustine!" Chris has a knack for trivia, and he calls it "unusable knowledge." He always takes opportunities to get involved with other people, which also helps take his mind off the hard work in therapy. After a good half hour, Chris was back on the mat and it was time to transfer back to the chair and back to the mat a few more times before therapy ended for the day.

At 5 p.m., when therapy ended, Chris and Carrie, JD and his mom Jackie, and Will and his mom Kim all planned to meet at a restaurant in the inner harbor along with my sister and my husband, and Roxanne and Tucker, who my sister and I introduced to Carrie and Chris several years prior. Of course, Carrie made a reservation so that four wheelchairs could be around the table along with eight other people. The four boys, while not really close friends, have something in common that has brought them together. They all have had spinal cord injuries that caused paralysis.

JD dove from a bridge into a river in Arkansas. Luckily there was an EMS person on a canoe who came to his rescue. When I asked JD about the accident, he said he didn't regret diving first even though it was his friend's idea to dive into the river, not his. They both could have dove at the same time, or his buddy could have gone first and been the one injured. But that was not the case, and amazingly, JD is okay with that. His friend, on the other hand, felt very guilty about encouraging JD to dive.

Will, who was in a car accident and suffers from SCI with Central Cord Syndrome, said over lunch that he would like to go surfing or do something crazy because what else does he have to lose. He goes to college and lives in a house with three friends, with a caregiver attending to his needs. Tucker, who also dove into a sandbar like Chris, has become a painter using talents he had not put to use before his accident; he is selling his paintings to help pay for therapy.

Like Chris, who is attending Harvard and has gotten into photography, all three of these young men have not let the tragedy of their accident ruin their lives. It was apparent to me that day how important their relationships are—between patients, between patient and PT, between patient and caregiver, as well as among the caregivers themselves. A network is formed when people are placed in similar situations. People who would not otherwise have had relationships become support systems for each other. Being able to bounce an idea off someone else, ask for advice, or maybe even share some sorrows helps the healing process.

CHAPTER 21

Life Is Good

When one door closes another door opens; but we so often look so
long at the closed door, that we don't see the ones which open for us.
—ALEXANDER GRAHAM BELL[29]

Coming back home to the familiar after being away is always a good feeling. I really do love being home. It brings a sense of normalcy. The intensity of the therapy lessens, and we get back into a routine: therapy at Gaylord, work at Access Independence, home in the afternoon to study and work on assignments for Harvard. Mom, Dad, Matt, and I are all around in a normal family kind of way. But somehow I yearn for the hard work of the therapy that keeps my muscles alive and awake at Kennedy Krieger.

When I felt a sensation in my foot and quads during pool therapy that had been forgotten since my accident, a surge of excitement and energy shot through me. As a result, my doctor put me on a ground-breaking medicine for MS patients. It is possible with the medicine to have enhanced sensations. After ten days, nothing had changed but

I remained optimistic. As with any medicine, there are side effects, one of which is low blood pressure—something I experienced in the early days after my accident. I got nauseous and had headaches. This was not a welcomed side effect, but one I was willing to deal with for a period of time if it meant getting more feeling back in my limbs.

There was no more IPA tasting with Kevin while taking the medicine. Drinking alcohol can enhance negative side effects and bring on seizures. You've got to give up something to gain results! After three months, my doctor decided the medicine was not having any positive effects and told me to stop taking it. I gave it a shot, and it didn't help. However, I am confident there will be other medicines and new technology invented that I can try as time goes on.

After three brief weeks at home, we were off to Shepherd Center in Atlanta once again, and Matt was back to Siena College for his senior year. Dad would be solo. I often think about how it is for him coming home from work, where his focus is paying for my health care, to an empty, quiet house. After another five weeks at Shepherd, it was really good to be home again for the Christmas holidays. Despite the therapy at Shepherd not going quite the way I expected, I was feeling good, my family was good, life was good—we were all in a good place. If it had been several years prior, I would have been upset with the outcome. This time, however, I had so much else going for me in my life that the therapy issues didn't affect me too much. Yes, I wanted to get every bit out of my rehab as possible, but right now I was able to move forward despite not getting the support I'd hoped for. Instead of making gains at Shepherd, I was taking leaps in my life as a person.

So many positive things happened that year: I was hired by Access Independence. Instead of working fifteen hours per week for the state, I began working twenty hours and getting paid as an employee. We hired two caregivers so that my mom could work part-time. I enrolled in the Harvard Extension School, initially working toward a degree in psychology with a minor in law. I'm on an upward track. My physical therapy, while still hugely important, was not first and foremost in my mind every day. I was excited to go to work, and eager to take challenging classes and do my schoolwork. I was encouraged and enthusiastic about new opportunities and the potential in my life. My outlook was positive.

Life is good. It might sound crazy, but I wouldn't be in as good a place if it weren't for my accident. Some doors have closed for me, but so many others have opened right before my eyes. I realized this more than ever when I attended a wedding for my freshman-year swim team captain. Due to my situation, my parents came to South Carolina with me. They didn't attend the wedding but stayed in a hotel nearby, which was also where I would be staying. They expected me to get a ride back to the hotel later that night by some of my old college buddies who were also on the swim team.

When I called my mom to pick me up at 8:30 p.m., her first response was, "What's the matter?" She knew instantly that something was wrong just by the tone in my voice. Nothing terrible was wrong; my buddies had been drinking and really couldn't attend to my needs. They were just having a good time getting together, having not seen each other in a long while, but I needed to be cathed. It was like they just picked up where they left off in college, instead of picking up where they are in life now. I can't go back to the way it was before.

I'm in a different place. It's ironic that while I've grown up faster than my college buddies, I can't completely take care of myself. At the wedding, they were still in the college party stage and didn't realize that they let me down that night. They didn't understand—nor did they really need to understand—what it's like to be dependent on someone else. There were no hard feelings. The good news is my chair did not define me that night. For my buddies I was the same Chris they knew in college: the partier, the risk taker, the fun-loving person who never missed an event. Reality is, though, that my needs and my life are very different now. It will never be the same again because I have grown in so many ways through this experience. As a result, I am a stronger person, a wiser person, a better-rounded person than I ever was before.

CHAPTER 22

Once a Sailor,
Always a Sailor

Sailing takes me away to where I've always heard it could be.
Just a dream and the wind to carry me.
And soon I will be free.[30]

We aren't home from Shepherd for more than a few months and we are off to Kennedy Krieger in Baltimore once again, this time for two weeks. Each time I return to a rehab facility, I have great expectations for myself and for those who will work with me. It's always great to see therapists and doctors I have worked with in the past. When one of the therapists commented, with tears in her eyes, how much stronger I am now than the last time she saw me, I felt like bouncing out of my chair to hug her. Her words make the hard work worth the effort.

These few weeks at Kennedy Krieger brought forth a lot of hope and strength. I felt closer to my before-accident self than ever when I had therapy using a sailing simulator called a VSail Trainer. I was able to navigate a dinghy on a virtual course as you would an actual sailboat. An electronic joystick acts like a tiller to control the rudder and steer the boat, and a mainsheet controls the sail. As I sat in the boat with the mainsheet in my right hand and used the joystick with my left hand, I felt like I was out on the water. My sailing instincts kicked in immediately, and I forgot for a moment that I am paralyzed and that I was not on the water. An adrenalin rush came over me as I jibed the boat without giving my therapist any warning. The boat literally jibed from one side to the other with an abrupt motion that made bystanders jump back. I just chuckled when my therapist hollered out, "What happened?" The therapist, who was not an educated sailor, actually learned from me as I virtually sailed around a course, smiling all the way. Hopefully this will lead me to Baltimore Harbor when I return to Kennedy Krieger during the outdoor sailing months.

Kennedy Krieger launched a pilot study using a Virtual Sailing Vsail Trainer with SCI patients in 2011. This study came under the direction of Dr. Albert Recio, who believes that recreational experiences have a huge impact on the quality of life for an SCI patient. The Virtual Sailing VSail Trainer is the first sailing simulator available for people with paralysis. The stationary, motorized sailboat cockpit features specialized software that enables patients to navigate the boat around a virtual course in the same way as an actual sailboat in the water. Electronic sensors give the participant real-time feedback that matches their movements and allows them to control wind strength and water conditions. The results of the study showed that

- all participants demonstrated rapid and substantial improvement in their sailing scores.

- all patients showed a significant positive increase in overall quality of life, including increased self-confidence and sense of accomplishment.
- following completion of the training program, all subjects were able to successfully sail and perform specific maneuvers on the water at a sailing center in Baltimore.[31]

While at Kennedy Krieger, I also *walked* on what is essentially an elliptical machine with support from my therapists. It was an awesome feeling to actually see my legs moving. As with the FES bike, my feet were locked into pedals, and stimulation pads or electrodes then stimulated the muscles to get them to move. I also did something new where I was supported by an above-ground harness, which went better than in the past. I had electrodes on my spine and my stomach that stimulated my legs while the therapist helped me move the muscles in my quads. Then I'd be in the pool for an hour, which might sound relaxing but is not at all. I hadn't been in the pool as much at home due to working and taking classes, so the advances there were not as great despite feeling stronger overall from past visits to Kennedy Krieger. In the pool, I worked with some different core stability exercises for back and abs which I now needed to take back home with me to maintain the growth. Having worked with some new therapists and new techniques, I left Kennedy Krieger feeling inspired and hopeful.

CHAPTER 23

I'm Good

As 2016 began, I felt thankful. I was healthy and getting stronger every day. I was in a good place unlike the many people with SCI that get sick often, get sores, reflux, and so many other illnesses or side effects. Continuing online classes with Harvard Extension School, and working thirty hours a week—I was in a really good place. I just had to keep it moving every day.

Now it was Kennedy Krieger every few months. My new goal for being back at Kennedy Krieger was to participate in the adaptive sailing in Baltimore Harbor. I envisioned myself out on a small dinghy with the real water of the harbor surrounding me, feeling the breeze in my face, and thinking only of sailing the boat. I yearned to be free of the fear of not being in control, and what better way to achieve that than by doing something I am still passionate about.

I know what dangers sailors can encounter out on the water when a storm comes up out of nowhere, when the weather is in control and the sailor is not. Because I know these things, I have a fear of getting into a situation that I can't manage. For me to be in a boat that capsized would be devastating. What would I do? Who would help me? These thoughts go through my head. When they do, I try very hard to shut them out. Perhaps the only way to get rid of the fear is to conquer it.

Meanwhile, we had hired two new caregivers, a change that took time getting used to. It was kind of weird having someone other than my mom with me all the time. Not to be snobby, but I don't want to be talking with caregivers; I just want them there to help me when I need them. I'm not trying to be selfish, but chitchat drives me nuts. I might be concentrating on an online course and my caregiver asks me if I need anything, and I lose my train of thought. My goal is to do as much as I can on my own. If I need help, I will ask. It took a while to get used to having caregivers other than my mom, but that didn't last long.

Things were going well with Mom working and with my job and school. She didn't have to do as much for me anymore, but there were times still when I'd rather she did things for me than someone else. One morning when my first caregiver arrived, and it was time to brush my teeth and get out the door, Mom was standing right there in the kitchen. She could have brushed my teeth, which I suggested with a look, but she gave me that look back that said, "Not a chance, Christopher. You have a caregiver now." So the caregiver brushed my teeth, not the same I might add. It's a transition I have to get used to if I want to be independent from home.

Truth be told, we were in a routine and it was kind of nice. My mom really didn't have to hang with me all the time, and it was good being just the two of us. Matt was back at school and Dad was gone a lot. While the holidays were busy, fun, and great to have everyone home, the quiet is always welcome. When everyone's home, Mom feels like she has to entertain everyone, have enough food in the house, worry about what's for dinner, keep the house neat. It's a revolving door of family and friends.

Selfishly, I get annoyed when she can't focus on me. It's frustrating when everyone is around and I have to wait to do what I want *when* I want to do it. When it's just the two of us, we are in sync and there is less pressure. She doesn't really have to worry about me, but she always knows when I need a drink, have to go to the bathroom, or need something. She can go about doing her own thing around the house, make phone calls, chat with friends, and relax a little between helping me. It just works.

PART IV

A BEACON OF
STRENGTH

He helps us in all our troubles, so that we are able to help others
who have all kinds of troubles, using the same help that we
ourselves have received from God.
(2 CORINTHIANS 1:4 GNB)

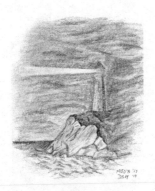

The lighthouse is a beacon of strength among the calm and the turbulent seas for boats navigating their way. While Chris is unaware, his words and actions now strengthen, comfort, and navigate others to find their way. Many of Chris's family and friends reached out to me with stories of how he has impacted their lives.

CHAPTER 24

Putting Life in Perspective

Alecia

I met Chris in February 2014 after my brother was admitted to the Shepherd Center following a serious car accident that left him paralyzed from the waist down. My brother is only a few years older than Chris, and being faced with a new life, although he was lucky to have it, brought heartache, uncertainty, anger, and depression. Situations like this take a toll on a family in ways no one can expect. It's no exaggeration when I say meeting Chris and his family was, and still is, a beacon of hope in a very difficult time. Chris's constant positive and friendly demeanor are what attract people to him; his vulnerability, honesty, and hopefulness are what make him an inspiration.

Not knowing what to say or how to treat a young man whose life had been flipped upside down, my family often turned to Chris for answers and encouragement. He reiterated that things would get better; he explained why things would get harder first; he shared lessons of what helped him through his toughest days; he offered his support the whole way. In a time when we worried things would never be the same again, he shed light on a brighter, better future. His gratitude for life and his family is infectious, and after being around him for ten minutes, people can't help but feel happy.

Chris has no doubt overcome innumerable odds physically and mentally, but the way he treats others, despite all he's gone through, and views the future is what pushes others to greatness for themselves. He is an example that perseverance, optimism, and hard work can not only change your own life, but the lives of those around you. I know my entire family will forever be grateful that Chris and his family crossed our path in life.

My family and I are very close with four kids, each two years apart, and the six of us spend a lot of time together, so my brother Shaun's accident and recovery became our priority from day one. We all flew or drove to Charleston, South Carolina, where Shaun was living, the morning after the accident, then traveled together to Pittsburgh where he was in the hospital for about six weeks. After that, he was admitted to the Shepherd Center. I felt oddly blessed because I was living in Atlanta, and Shepherd was literally a mile down the road from me.

From February to July 2014, Shaun went to physical therapy daily and met quite a few guys around his age—all from different backgrounds and different accidents, but all wanting to get better. Ironically, Shaun and Chris both had gone to the College of Charleston but didn't know each other as Shaun is four years older than Chris, so they bonded immediately. My mom, who was living with Shaun here in Atlanta, met Carrie through the gym at Shepherd, and they quickly became friends.

On every level, Carrie is just as inspiring to my family as Chris. At the time we thought, *Carrie and Chris were in a similar boat, just ahead of us.* My mom leaned on Carrie for support and guidance of what was to come, and they became very good friends. Carrie and Chris were incredibly welcoming, friendly, fun, and thoughtful. Many emotions that I didn't even know existed surfaced during this time. The fact that Carrie and Chris had been through it all a year or so before us led us to look up to them for hope. They were and still are this very close, optimistic family who values their time together and sees the future as limitless. At the time, that was not something my family and I could comprehend. Their friendship to our family was more than friendship; it was hope, support, inspiration, and reassurance. Their kindness never wavered, even when they, or we, were having a difficult day or week. At times when I wasn't sure how our family would make it through this, I looked to them, especially Chris, and saw that no matter what, there is always something worth fighting for.

Chris inspires me personally too. He looks at life and sees no boundaries; if there are boundaries, he is convinced not to let them get in his way of greatness. Since meeting Chris, seeing and hearing what he's been through, I will admit that his attitude and perseverance cross my mind daily. Sometimes it's in small ways like pushing myself to the next level at the gym or taking the stairs because I can. Sometimes it's in bigger ways like using what I learned from Chris and my brother to get involved in disability support groups at work and networking with other individuals with disabilities. Most of the time, it's just taking a step back from life to look at everything I have and feeling grateful.

Chris, like the rest of us, could look at his own life and find negatives, but since I've known him, he's never done that. He inspired me to appreciate life, work with what I'm given, and make the most out of every situation.

Kiera

I met Chris and Carrie at the Promotion Gym at Shepherd Center in February 2014. My son had a spinal cord injury from a car accident in December of 2013, leaving him paralyzed from the waist down. It turned our world upside down and left me struggling and wondering how I would cope. And I'm just the "Mom," not the one living in his shoes.

I noticed this handsome young man on an exercise bike, his wheelchair on one side, his mom on the other. He was working so hard and smiling a big grin at the same time. He and his mom shared words and laughter. He had on a College of Charleston shirt, which is where my son had graduated from a year earlier. I introduced myself to him and learned that he went to C of C and was an athlete on the swim/dive team there. I also learned of his accident two years prior and that he was now a quadriplegic. And that is where his handicap ends.

All I can say is *wow!* After getting to know Chris (and Carrie), he blew me away with his sensitivity, his maturity, his helpfulness and guidance. Not once did I see pity or helplessness. I saw him helping others cope. My son and I sat back and wondered, "How does he do it? How does he stay positive and happy mentally and work so incredibly hard physically toward recovering and walking again?" Chris has a gift of helping others while he works so hard at helping himself. He is an inspiration. He is a pleasure to be around. We are lucky to have met him. He also has a great family and support system, and a mom who is an angel, who helped me to cope. And he has that beautiful grin that spreads across his face!

Shaun

I just don't have the same determination that Chris has even though his injury is worse than mine. In December of 2013, I was a passenger in my buddy's truck when it rolled. I was thrown out the window only to become paralyzed from the waist down. Like Chris, my life changed instantly. I went from athlete to paraplegic, but unlike Chris, I felt pretty sorry for myself. My family was at my beck and call at first, but being a paraplegic not a quad made it possible for me to be somewhat independent eventually. My family gave me a great deal of moral support. Fortunately, my dad was able to afford the best rehabilitation center, where I met Chris O'Brien.

When I arrived at Shepherd, one of the therapists introduced us and we connected right away. We had both gone to the College of Charleston in South Carolina and had a lot in common. I was a D1 lacrosse player and Chris was a D1 swimmer for the college. Both of us had an identity of "athlete". Despite my accident, I was fortunate to graduate in 2012 with a bachelor's degree in computer science, whereas Chris would not be able to go back to the C of C after his accident. Currently, I work part-time out of my home with a blue chip company, and I live with a few other college grads. I'm lucky that I can do my job now from my house and live pretty independently since I left Shepherd. I can use my hands, so it's quite different from being a quad. Even so, I'm still not the person I want to be.

At Shepherd, I drew from Chris's cheerfulness. His injury was far more severe than mine, but he was far happier than me, and I knew it. I was even a bit jealous of Chris. He was always happy and smiling. There were a handful of times we'd go out with our moms and my sister. Sometimes I wouldn't even want to be there, and I'd have to check in with myself and think, *Why can't I be more upbeat like Chris?* Being around Chris and seeing how he carried himself was an inspiration. When you're around people who are fighting paralysis, words kind of lose their meaning. People repeat the same thing: "Keep at it," "You're doing great," "Stay positive." Their words become diluted after a while, but being with Chris was real.

When we first met at the gym, Chris invited me over to his apartment for dinner. We both lived in housing near the gym. I went over to Chris's place with my brother and sister. My mom was out of town, but we would have many other evenings together with Carrie and Chris. I didn't really know anybody at Shepherd, so it was nice to have Chris there. He and Carrie were both quick to be friends and wanted to help. It was comforting to have them there to support me. We sat around sharing our experiences and had a fun time despite my not wanting to be there at first. We never really gave each other advice; it was more by example. We talked about where we were in terms of rehab. And we continued to see each other working hard at the gym there.

Being a paraplegic is a lonely injury. Feeling like a victim, I continue to struggle every day. My family has given me lots of moral support, but no one can completely understand what it's like unless they've been there. The biggest challenge for me is accepting my new identity even though I can get most every place I want. I was an athlete and one of the best in my sport. Then to accept this new identity was, and still is, a mental game. It is where many paraplegics and quadriplegics fall into depression.

I keep telling myself that if Chris can be positive, then I can too. When you see someone like Chris working hard, it gives you the motivation to push forward and never give up. Chris and I still text each other, and I've seen him a few other times. Perhaps with time, a mix of Chris's determination and perseverance will give me enough to reboot my own determination and outlook on life.

Greg

Have you ever had a friend who thinks and acts like you do? One where you know what the other is thinking or about to say even before they speak. One who makes you a better person because of who they are? Chris O'Brien is that friend. We met in August 2010 as swim teammates at the College of Charleston and instantly became best friends. We turned best friends, then into brothers. Both tall, lanky, goofy kids who were going to be on the Division 1 swim team together wondering where we would fit in. Both of us couldn't kick if our lives depended on it, and together we had a blast during kick sets looking at each other in our respective lanes thinking, *What the heck are we doing, and how did we get here?*

Not only did we swim together, but because we think so much alike, we hung out together, relied on each other, and at times got into trouble together. He was my go-to for everything. Chris and I both have a bit of a wild side. Neither of us will ever forget "Balcony Day" when a bunch of us hoisted beer into our dorm room, which was obviously illegal. Chris was hanging off the second-floor balcony to retrieve the case while I was holding onto his legs praying he wouldn't fall. Not very intelligent, but we were just a bunch of crazy college kids releasing our energies after a successful swim season. It's hard for me to think back to some of the outlandish, dangerous stuff we survived in college and then imagine him paralyzed after a simple dive in the ocean.

Most kids have comic book heroes that they look up to, but that usually phases out with age. Well, I am lucky to still have one. Chris. Chris O'Brien is *my* superhero. His accident only made us closer. Sure, we weren't in the same area, and he wasn't coming back to school, but he was still with me, everywhere and in everything I did. Everything the team and I did from that point forward was for our brother, Chris. We fed off his hard work and determination, and he fed off our success when he would come to the meets and watch that hard work pay off.

Chris was an active volunteer firefighter, as I am now. He talked proudly of his training and being part of the brotherhood. I became a volunteer firefighter in part because of Chris, and I love it every bit as much as he did. To be a firefighter you have to be willing to sacrifice your life for another. You have to be willing to take a risk and not fear what could happen. You have to trust in yourself and in your brothers completely. All these characteristics describe Chris and who he is, even more so today. Chris will always be my inspiration, my motivation, and my determination. When he takes that first step, I will be right there with him, if not physically, then in spirit.

Patrick

When Chris walked onto the pool deck at the College of Charleston for the first time, I saw a tall, athletic-looking kid with an air of confidence. As a senior and the captain of the team, I had heard we had a freshman walk-on, which is not always ideal. Despite being a walk-on to the team, which means working harder than anyone else to qualify, Chris was goal driven from day one. He stood out among the freshmen, who were usually a bit immature and quick to goof around. Chris knew he wasn't a star on the team, and he didn't let that stop him. In fact, it pushed him harder. What made Chris shine was his work ethic, no-nonsense mentality, and his maturity. He was determined to be a Division 1 swimmer with a record.

Most seniors don't choose to hang out with freshmen even if they are teammates. There's quite a difference between a wet-behind-the-ears newbie and a senior, even a sophomore or a junior for that matter. It was different with Chris. We bonded instantly, and he hung out with me and three juniors from the team after practice and on weekends. On an occasional Saturday night, we'd go out and have a good time, sometimes too good a time. Even so, Chris would be up and ready for practice on Sunday morning. Chris and I not only shared a common interest in swimming, but sailing too. We got out on the water a few times, and even though Chris started sailing as a teenager, I quickly learned that he was a far better sailor than me. He was comfortable on a boat like he was in his own skin. He knew how to read the wind, and he was teaching me how to sail faster while I coached him how to swim faster.

Swimming was hard for Chris. He struggled with his kick just like he did in high school. He still couldn't quite get his legs and feet to do what they were supposed to do. The coach gave him some extra exercises to do at the gym to strengthen his legs in hopes of improving his kick, which would ultimately improve his speed. He hated doing squats, but Chris would be in the weight room lifting, training, doing extra squats to strengthen his legs, going the extra mile when everyone else was done for the day.

It wasn't surprising when Chris broke his record and won at the championships that year, it was expected. That win put him in a different league of swimmers, and his future as a D1 swimmer for the College of Charleston was bright. The team respected Chris and his determination. Everyone admired him and loved having him on the team. So it was a shock to all of us when we heard about Chris's accident. Initially, we didn't have all the facts and were just putting pieces of information together. The more we learned, the more we felt the reality, and the more we felt the devastation knowing that Chris would not be coming back to the College of Charleston to swim with the team. In fact, Chris would not be coming back at all. We mourned *our* loss.

After graduating from the College of Charleston, I went to Louisiana State University for grad school and then came back to Charleston to start my career as an environmental consultant. Life was busy, so I didn't see Chris until my wedding, four years after he became paralyzed. I was very excited when Chris responded that he would attend my wedding, but I wondered nervously what it was going to be like to see him after all this time. I wondered how he would look, how he would seem. I had spoken to Chris on the phone a bunch of times, and he always seemed positive. Was it a facade? Would he really have the same positive outlook on life when I saw him in person?

My wedding day arrived. I stood proudly at the altar, and when my eyes met Chris's, I saw the same spark and smiling face. Goosebumps covered my arms and a wave of emotion caught my breath. Finally, at the reception, I was able to catch up with him. It was like old times, and I didn't even notice his chair. He was the same person I knew in college, a person who wanted to hang out with his buddies, tell jokes, laugh, and live life. Later, I thought about how someone else in Chris's shoes might let their chair define who they had become, feel sorry for themselves, and ask why me. Not Chris. Every time I talk to him, he's excited about his rehabilitation and what he has accomplished.

As far as I'm concerned, Chris has accomplished more in his life already than most do in a lifetime. I am inspired by him every day. When I have a bad day and get down on myself, my mind goes to Chris. How can I get discouraged and give up when Chris is encouraged and fighting for his life every day without a complaint? Chris O'Brien is an anomaly.

Gina

My twin sons, Keith and Daniel, played baseball and soccer with Matt for as long as I can remember, and they are still friends today. My husband and I sat on many sidelines with the O'Briens but did not get to know Chris well until after his accident.

When I did get to know Chris, he inspired me on many levels. The first thing that comes to mind is how he has handled the cards he's been dealt with such maturity for a young man. He has adapted to his current limitations, but not been defined by them. He has such determination to reach the next level of his ability and recovery and faces each task with both grit and positivity. I have no doubt that Chris will continue to face life's challenges head-on, and make progress each and every day.

The next thing that comes to mind is Chris's sense of humor. From the time of his accident until now, he has used his humor to put people at ease. Recently, someone asked me if it was difficult and sad to see this young man in a wheelchair. Never have I felt sad after seeing Chris; quite the opposite. Every time I have left a visit with Chris, I have felt truly uplifted. He is an amazing young man who is engaged with his family and friends. He always asks how my sons are doing and wants to hear the details of their lives. We have shared so many laughs about the situations we all get ourselves into.

I am inspired by his determination to continue his education and impressed that he was accepted to Harvard. Obviously, they saw the special qualities we all know Chris possesses. Again, I have no doubt he will be successful in whatever work path he chooses. I am inspired by Chris's friends and the outpouring of love and support they have given. It goes hand-in-hand; to receive that kind of true friendship, you need to have given it. Today we hear so many negative things about the Millennials, about how they are so entitled, focused on social media, selfish. But the group of young people who travel in Chris's path are all positive examples of caring, compassion, and commitment to their friendships.

I am also truly inspired by Carrie, Paul, and Matt. Chris's accident changed not only his life, but that of his family. Each of them has found their role in Chris's recovery and taken the reins and run with them. They are all so positive and determined to support Chris and live their lives to the fullest extent as a family.

Some lessons I have learned from watching the journey of Chris and the O'Brien family that I now share with my own boys are: First, adapt to what life throws at you, big or small, and face it with a positive attitude, determination, and humor. Second, friendship is one of the most important parts of life. Always strive to be the best friend you can be. If you are a good friend, you will always have someone to share the good times with and support you through the difficult ones.

Andrea

Conflicting feelings make me uneasy at times. I grieve for the loss of my day-to-day friendship with one of my best friends, and I feel guilty about it at the same time. Carrie still is one of my closest friends, but life is different now. I wonder if Carrie, in some way, mourns her old life and the change in some of her friendships. Some friends have come, and some have gone. There are people Carrie didn't think would be there for her that rose to the occasion, and others who sadly and unexpectedly stopped coming around.

It's challenging and confusing to lose a relationship with a good friend, for whatever reason. Don't get me wrong. I haven't lost my friendship, it has just changed. For so many years, I'd call up Carrie to see if she wanted to go to the gym or for a walk, and that was what we would do. Then Chris had the accident. Suddenly Carrie's focus was Chris, all Chris, which is completely understandable. But I missed the times when we'd just walk and catch up, talk about ourselves, our families, what our plans were for the weekend…life. Looking back, friendship seemed so simple then.

When Chris had the accident, I went to the house daily to help Carrie, and what always amazed me was her optimistic attitude. I would help however needed. In the beginning, it was tasks like assisting Chris out of his chair and into the bathroom for a shower. Then it was back to his bed, feeding him, and making sure he was comfortable. We were kind of winging it, doing the best we could, but Carrie always seemed like she knew what she was doing.

One day Carrie bluntly said, "We are done crying about Chris. We are picking up the pieces and we are moving on." I was amazed by this matter-of-fact statement. The truth is that she never did cry again over Chris's accident, at least in front of others. She was stoic and faced the issue the way she faces any conflict: strong, with a positive attitude, and in control. Sometimes I want her to call me, cry about it, and tell me what's going on down deep inside her heart. If it were me, I'd be crying all the time and looking for sympathy. But Carrie is not like me. I know I wouldn't be strong like Carrie has been while taking care of her oldest son, who went from D1 swimmer to quadriplegic in a matter of minutes.

Even more amazing was Chris's attitude. He wasn't sulking or complaining or wondering why this had happened to him. The first time I went to see Chris in the hospital after the accident, I kept to small talk because *I* was nervous. Chris, on the other hand, was relaxed and pleasant. He was chatty as usual and even stopped a conversation and said, "Oh, how was your trip to Greece?" I was amazed by this and still today can't believe that he's so upbeat all the time. None of Carrie's friends can imagine themselves in her shoes. We've all talked about it. They are both unique people with the strongest faith I've ever known.

The first time Carrie came back from Gaylord after the accident to get some things, she looked exhausted, but she said point-blank, "We are not going to even entertain the idea that Chris won't walk again, but I'm withdrawing him for the year from the university." I think we all thought that since he had bruised, not severed, his spinal cord, he would be back to walking soon. We all thought that once Chris got down to Shepherd, he'd recover more quickly.

The reality is that Chris jumped from having one year of college under his belt to adulthood. He had to come to grips with his accident and spent more time with adults who could take care of him. He missed those last few wonder years of his youth. It used to be when we'd go over there, the boys would all be running around playing football outside. But now he's sitting around with the adults talking knowledgeably and maturely about the world news, his progress, and it's like he's one of the adults. Chris has gained a lot of strength in his life from his disability and has had to grow up before his time.

Kim

I only got to know Chris after the accident. Chris was always on the periphery when Matt and my son Brendan played baseball for Trumbull Little League. I remember one of the first times going over to the O'Briens' house when they returned from Gaylord and were settling in at home. The reality of the situation became immensely apparent when I excitedly took some occupational therapy stuff from school out of my bag—white boards, large crayons, large kindergarten pencil, and so forth—only to learn he couldn't hold onto even these items. Chris kind of shrugged it off and said, "Thanks. I'll be able to use those soon." My stomach sank, and I felt uneasy, wishing I could have helped.

Chris has touched all our lives. People who don't even know Chris are inspired by him. He did a favor for a family friend, a man who suffers from depression and anxiety and had some time on his hands. When he asked Carrie how he could help, Carrie told him they needed a table for Chris to do his stretching on, so he set to work, taking his mind off his own worries, and made the table. Chris actually gave this man a feeling he needed at a time when he was down.

Before his accident, Chris was in the best physical shape of his life. Girls were in awe of him, and Chris was at an all-time high. So for my sons and many of the other boys they grew up with, who completely admired and looked up to Chris, it was disbelief when they saw him after the accident. It was a harsh reality to see Chris and to think of him never walking again. After spending time together, though, they realized that Chris is the same person he was before.

They see that Chris doesn't want his chair to define him. For those of us who have known him his whole life, this is the absolute truth.

CHAPTER 25

Coach Mike

━━━━━

The potential of the average person is like a huge ocean unsailed,
a new continent unexplored, a world of possibilities waiting to
be released and channeled toward some great good.
—BRIAN TRACY[32]

I started coaching Chris when he was swimming for Trumbull Pisces at the age of twelve or so. Chris was young, had a smile on his face, and I knew he was a special kind of kid. Everybody loved Chris. From an early age he was the big man on campus. Our coach/swimmer relationship was good. I've never coached a kid with as much raw potential as Chris. He was tall and a great athlete, even if he says otherwise. Chris swam fast with his upper body. I remember saying, "If you ever figure out how to kick, we'll have something here." One day when he did kick the way I taught him, he took the ball and ran with it.

In practice day to day I reminded Chris to do the best he could do. I pushed him hard, and in return he pushed me to be the best

147

coach I could be. As with most teens, Chris usually had his own plan, so he needed to be motivated intrinsically. Once he realized that he needed to follow directions and trust me, he came around. Chris was a true sprinter. Typically, sprinters are more independent because they are swimming an individual race. The sprint is not as much about strategy and mechanics, but about speed. A sprinter just races as hard and fast as they can.

Chris's strength was swimming 50- and 100-meter freestyle. He could swim in an Individual Medly (IM) team relay, which included butterfly, backstroke, breaststroke, and his swimming the freestyle leg, but individual sprinting was his thing. Coaches always have a great bond with sprinters because it is such an intense race for both. When you watch a sprint, it's a beautiful race. Chris and I had many talks about what he could do if he set his mind to winning, and once he got to high school the word *determination* became intrinsic. He made the word his own.

Chris had talent that he didn't always see, but he was around positive people, and so many people were encouraging him to do his best even when he wanted to quit. Once Chris made up his own mind to put 100 percent into his swimming, he soared and reached goals we had set that he never believed he could reach. Initially, I had mixed feelings about Chris going to the College of Charleston and facing the rigors of the swim team on his own. I knew if he found the strength in himself and had a coach who believed in him, he could do it, and he absolutely did. His determination to win was evident in the end when Chris finished first place at the CCSA in his 100-meter freestyle. His last race at the C of C, when he broke his own record, was very symbolic of who he is and his perseverance that is evident today.

Chris's life has been preparation for where he is now. Perhaps this is all part of God's plan. God took a person like Chris, who has a very strong character and comes from a strong family, to share a life message with others: life doesn't always go as planned, but you have to work your hardest, do the best you can, and live your life to its fullest no matter what lemons it brings. The diving accident has actually allowed Chris to vault. He has had an impact on so many people in a positive way: my high school swimmers, my wife's University of Bridgeport gymnasts, friends, people he meets along the way— the numbers are huge. This accident, despite not being what anyone wanted for Chris or his family, has opened up a whole new world of opportunities.

No one really filled me in on the extent of Chris's injury and exactly what had happened. So when he rolled his wheelchair onto the pool deck one afternoon during practice, I got a huge lump in my throat and chills ran down my spine. He was wearing his favorite gray half-zipper sweatshirt and a C of C hat backwards just like always. Trying to swallow, I thought to myself, *The last thing I'm going to do here is cry.* I was thinking, *Can I touch him? Am I going to hurt him?* But Chris had this huge smile on his face like he was taking care of me. He simply said, "Hey, Coach, how's practice going today? What are we working on?"

It was like any other day. There was no woe is me. I leaned down, grabbed him, and hugged him; his body was much slighter than I remembered. From the moment I saw his expression, though, I knew Chris would be okay. I asked how he was doing. He said, "I can't sit around and sulk or have a bad day. It is what it is." I realized then that anyone can learn from Chris's message. So I asked him if he wanted to help coach, and he agreed. He worked with the sprinters for a season, talking to these kids like a confident coach. When Chris went to Shepherd Center in Georgia after that, he sent a video of himself doing physical therapy in the pool, and I showed it to the team. They all hollered and cheered; obviously he made an impact on their lives too.

My job now is to always be there as a friend and to support Chris in his new life goals. I have a clear responsibility to teach Chris's message to my swimmers: remain determined and never give up. We will always have a coach/swimmer relationship, but it has gone beyond that time. Now I see a young man I coached show me that what I taught him, he has taken to an even higher level. When I asked Chris to talk to the Trumbull Pisces swimmers about his accident and its impact on his life, he was unsure about what to say to them. Once he began, though, he was a very natural speaker, telling his story with ease.

Later, I asked him to talk to my swimmers in New Canaan. With the help of his brother, Chris put together a presentation that would impact these swimmers' lives more than he would ever know. Today I am coaching him in a different way—about presentation and communication skills. Chris still loves to be coached, and it is such a rush for both of us to work together again.

CHAPTER 26

Meg

Everyone faces challenges. I am not alone.

A typical fifth-grade day begins with a Teacher Education Association meeting in the library, writing morning announcements for my students, getting them started on morning routines before a sub arrives so I can head to my morning planning time, plus getting ready for a school-wide pep rally. It was a busy Friday morning when the secretary came down the hall to tell me I had a phone call. I looked up from demonstrating to the Student Council kids how to put a paw print on every student's hand before they walked into the pep rally and asked her if she could take a message. She said, "No. You need to take this call. He's going to be okay, but…" When I heard, "He's going to be okay," I thought of my sons, Billy and Peter, and my husband, Brian. Which one was hurt? All are such risk takers that it could have been any one of them.

"He got in a motorcycle accident," Denice said, which was when I knew that it was my husband, his second motorcycle accident in three years. I picked up the phone in the lounge and spoke to a nurse from St. Mary's Hospital in Waterbury who described Brian's motorcycle accident as horrific. My heart sank, and I could only think the worst. She informed me that Brian was in bad shape. He had some broken bones, and they weren't sure yet whether he could walk. She said that he was being put through tests to make sure everything else, such as his brain, was okay. What ran through my mind was his spine, his brain, his ability to walk.

Immediately, I thought about Chris. I wondered if Brian would be able to walk again, and of course I pictured the worst. As a teacher, you can't just leave twenty-four students to fend for themselves. Plans have to be put in place, and a substitute has to be available. But on that day, I rushed out of my classroom, leaving my student teacher to fend for herself, and began what would be a very long day, night, and many months ahead.

Every time Brian rode his motorcycle to work, I'd say, as I did that morning, "Be careful. I'm not ready to be a widow." I never wanted Brian to have a motorcycle in the first place. It has been a bone of contention. He'd already been in an accident three years prior where he was lucky enough to walk away. I had just gone through surgery on my neck for a fusion of C5-6 a few days earlier. I needed at least six weeks to recuperate, and now he was injured too. So, instead of calling me from the hospital, Brian called my son telling him about the accident and that he would need to be picked up once discharged.

When Billy didn't head to his summer job as a lifeguard that morning, saying he had something he had to do later, my instincts kicked in. I just knew something was wrong, and when I asked Billy to tell me the truth, he did. Later, Billy went to pick up his dad at the hospital and bring him home. Now Brian had to heal, and so did I. What a pathetic pair we were for the summer ahead. The good news was our boys were home to help out. The accident on September 25, 2015, was a completely different story.

On my way to St. Mary's Hospital, all I could think about was Chris O'Brien. Had my work with Chris prepared me for being a caregiver? I didn't know what to expect when I saw Brian. Was he paralyzed? Had his brain been injured? There were no answers yet. I arrived at the St. Mary's ER forty minutes later. The triage doctor was very matter-of-fact; no emotion, no feeling, just the facts. "Brian is in critical condition. We can't treat him here. We are sending him to Yale as soon as possible." As soon as possible turned into four hours later. While he was rolled out of St. Mary's on a gurney, I schlepped his bag of clothes, including his leather riding boots, a heavy leather jacket, a helmet, and the rest of his personal items to my car, which was parked down the street.

Meanwhile, Brian was taken to Yale by ambulance, arriving around 2 p.m. I drove my car and entered the ER, not knowing at the time that I would not leave that building for twenty-four hours. Brian was lying in the ER, hooked up to an IV, and in excruciating pain. He would be taken for a CAT scan, X-rays, ultrasounds, and many more tests over the next nine hours. When the doctor came to tell me the CAT scan of his brain came back normal, I burst into thankful tears. The X-rays confirmed that he had a broken hip and his femur was broken in two places. Brian also had several major lacerations to the left leg below the knee, leaving his leg dangling. When I first saw the lacerations, which looked like raw, bloody meat, I thought there was no possible way that anyone, even the most talented doctor, could put that leg back together. It looked like chopped beef and made my stomach turn.

Doctors, nurses, social workers, and the chaplain were in and out of the ER talking with us, giving us support. That was when I realized the severity of the situation. The pain was evident. Every time a nurse or doctor touched Brian's leg or moved it slightly, I could see the sheer pain on his face.

The next unexpected step was torture. Serious torture. The doctor explained that she had to drill a screw through the bone above his knee to hold the leg in place, all without anesthesia. There was no choice given the situation, and the next thing we knew the doctor had the drill in hand with a screw about ten inches long. She told Brian to brace himself because this was going to hurt like there's no tomorrow. While Brian is a firefighter and willing to run into a burning building to save someone, he has no stomach for blood, gore, or pain. Surprisingly, the doctor asked me to stay and hold his hand. I heard the drill start and watched as the doctor pushed the spiral screw through Brian's leg. The sound reminded me of the construction worker drilling drywall into our bathroom and sent a shiver up my spine. Brian held my hand so tight I seriously thought it might break. The screw entered Brian's flesh and began going deeper, the sound shrill and loud, the drill moving faster. When it hit the bone with a thud, Brian began to scream. Terror lit up his eyes, the pain going so deep, until he couldn't take it anymore and yelled, "Stop! Stop! Stop!"

"We are almost there," the doctor replied without emotion as she drilled just a bit further. The screw finally appeared on the other side of his leg. Brian gasped. In complete shock, his face was pale, pasty, and sweaty. The next task was to stabilize the leg with a metal gauge and rope until the surgeon was available for surgery, which would not be until 10 p.m. that night, fourteen hours after the accident.

For the next week, I'd be at the hospital from morning until night or after work until late when I'd go home to an empty house, aside from my crazy puppy, Gia. One night I arrived home at 9 p.m., not having eaten anything for dinner, exhausted from working until 5 and then being at the hospital until 8:30, to find Gia had shredded a bunch of my favorite books. One, ironically, was titled *The Book Thief*.

I literally sat down with my coat on and sobbed like a baby. During the stress of that week, I daily thought about Carrie and how she managed when Chris was in the hospital, in a halo brace, and learning that he was now a quadriplegic. I know she was exhausted and I know she cried, but she also said after a few days to me and other friends, "We are not going to cry anymore. It is what it is, and we need to pick up the pieces and move on." I would just wonder to myself how she did that, because I was a mess and couldn't stop crying.

After six days at Yale Medical, many tests, a high fever for several days, and then more tests, Brian was brought to a rehab facility closer to home. This was better for him because he would be in a healthier environment and begin therapy. For me it was better too, because I could go there after work, stay for a few hours, then be home in fifteen minutes. It was exhausting though, teaching all day long, feeling emotional, and wishing I could be with Brian. After work, I'd run home to let the dog out, then go to the rehab facility where I would help Brian however I could. I'd go home late, make my lunch for the next day, go through some paperwork, and sit with a glass of wine to watch the news. This was my only solace. Then each morning, I'd drag myself out of bed, give myself a pep talk, and trudge forward.

Brian came home ten days later, and I became his caregiver. Being a caregiver is no easy task, and I began feeling angry and resentful. My husband had bought a motorcycle when I was completely against it. I didn't stop him because then it would just be my fault on a sunny day when he wanted to go for a ride. My nightmare had become a reality for the second time. This time around, I was infuriated that now I had to stop my life to take care of him for something that didn't have to happen. This time around, the boys would be off at college and it would be me, just me. Again, I had a new respect for Carrie and any other caregiver.

Being a caregiver to a loved one is exhausting and trying on the relationship. After working all day, I'd come home and there would be a litany of things to be done: help Brian shower, change bandages, walk the dog, make dinner, make lunches for both of us, plan for my next day of teaching, and more. I felt like I was drowning, and some days I didn't want to get out of bed. I was tired and cranky and feeling guilty at the same time—such a conflict of emotions. On one hand, I was worried about Brian. On the other hand, I was livid. Expected feelings, I suppose, that come with worry and fear that a loved one will not fully recuperate. I can only imagine how the O'Brien family stayed so positive each day.

Everybody has something, something that makes their lives challenging. We don't always see it on the outside. People are good at hiding what's really going on in their lives behind the scenes. Sitting at church for the Thanksgiving mass, I became tearful when the priest read what parishioners had written about being thankful and realized that my *something* is no different from anyone else's something. If anything, mine is less but has felt like more, if that makes any sense.

People wrote, "I'm thankful for sobriety for two years," "I'm thankful for surviving cancer," "I'm thankful that my parents aren't fighting anymore," "I'm thankful for God saving my family from a fire." Then there was one that I could have written myself: "I'm thankful for God who saved my husband from a tragic accident and gave him strength to walk again." When I heard this I thought, *I am not alone.* How we deal with these events that alter our lives is a challenge each one of us faces differently.

I had spent weeks counting down the days for my boys to come home from college. Unable to visit them as planned during the fall, it had been three months since I'd last seen them, the longest I'd ever gone. The love I have for my boys can't be replaced by anything. So the moment Peter backed into the driveway and I heard the familiar sound of his truck, my heart raced and my eyes watered with tears of excitement. The hug from my six-foot-tall son flooded me with happiness. The next evening, Billy would back into the driveway and the same feelings would overcome me. His hugs would flood me again with joy. Seeing them hug each other and say "Hey bro" melted away all my feelings of loneliness. Having my young men under my roof is the best gift a mom could ask for over the holidays.

A few weeks before Thanksgiving, I was not in the mood to prepare a Thanksgiving feast for a large group, so I told my family it would just be Brian, the boys, and myself. I was feeling tired and just not in the mood to organize a celebration. Everyone was saddened by my lack of enthusiasm for the holidays, so I changed my mind and invited family. Since the holiday has always been about being with loved ones—aunts, uncles, cousins—I was happy with my decision.

On Thanksgiving morning, we headed over to the O'Briens' house for a short visit. There was Carrie with a houseful of friends visiting, laughing and having a great time. She continues to amaze me and be an inspiration. For me it's stressful to plan a get-together with family and friends, but she brings people together naturally and makes it look so simple.

That Thanksgiving night, a bunch of the kids who'd graduated from high school together and were now twenty-one gathered at a local bar. This included my son Billy and Carrie's son Matt. It was the first time they could all go out, meet at a bar, and have drinks legally. Thankfully, most of the kids use Uber and don't drive when drinking. Unfortunately, on this night, five of the young men were driving home from the bar when the car flipped, killing one of them and putting everything in perspective. The four who survived the accident would have to deal with this loss and the guilt for the rest of their lives. It could have been any one of our boys in that accident.

Again, I think of Carrie and Chris. Chris had an accident that changed his life, but he is alive, very much alive, and doing amazing things with his life. Losing a son or daughter is far more devastating than having a disabled son who is alive and loving life.

PART V

LIFE GOES ON

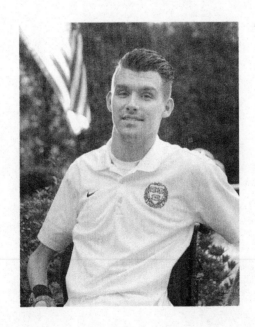

CHAPTER 27

What If?

Live as if you were to die tomorrow;
learn as if you were to live forever.
—MAHATMA GANDHI[33]

I n church recently the first reading was from the Book of Sirach and really struck a chord with me. "If you choose, you can keep the commandments, they will save you; if you trust in God, you too shall live; he has set before you fire and water; to which ever you choose stretch forth your hand."[34] Ironically, I have always chosen fire and water until now.

Have you ever played the "what if" game with yourself? Most people do on a regular basis. Sometimes I am afraid of simple things that could happen to me and start the "what if" game in my head. The honest truth is that I can get very nervous about the what-ifs in my life when I think too much about them. I have to listen to myself, then convince myself that life is too short to waste time thinking about what could happen but probably won't. Having once been a firefighter, I think about how I would get out of my house if there were a fire—certainly not by myself. As a probationary firefighter, I couldn't wait until I turned eighteen so I could run into a burning building and save a life.

Another big what-if is the thought of something happening to my mom, who takes care of me more than anyone else on a daily basis. Would I be able to live independently without her by my side? No. The reality is, she won't be able to care for me the way she does now forever. I picture myself driving a car someday, then I wonder what would happen if I were by myself and my body fell forward. What if I couldn't get myself back up off the steering wheel?

I've been longing to get back out on the water sailing, but as a sailor, I know what can happen when a squall comes out of nowhere. I've been there many times in big and small boats, and it can be very scary even to a seasoned sailor. The sky and ocean turn dark, the wind picks up speed, the waves swell, and your adrenalin kicks in. The crew has to act together, life jackets are thrown on quickly, the hatch is battened down, the mainsail is dropped, and all hands are on deck. What if that happened? What if I fell overboard? I wouldn't be able to get myself to safety without help. That thought really gives me nightmares. These not-so-little what-ifs are a result of my disabilities. When I think this way, I have to practice what I preach. It's a waste of time to worry about things I have no control over.

One night after a vivid dream about sailing again, I bumped into my old sailing friend Cliff Crowley at the Gaelic Club, and he told me about a sailing event at American Yacht Club for people who have been active sailors and now have disabilities. Cliff is the kind of person who doesn't take no for an answer. So when he asked about my interest, I hesitated, and he said, "Well, you are already signed up. It's the first weekend in June." I kind of chuckled but knew that Cliff was serious. I was going to sail again.

The Robie Pierce Regatta has been around for about ten years. Sailors with different disabilities come from all over to sail on Ideal 18s that have been adapted to their needs: blindness, paraplegics, amputees, and quadriplegics like me. It turns out I had the most severe disability of the sailors on the eighteen boats that were rigged for the regatta. Each boat had two disabled bodies and one able-bodied on board. Cliff would be the able-bodied sailor, which made me feel very secure. He has sailed in at least six Bermuda Races, has earned many awards including the "Storm Trysail" patch, and was the person who really taught me how to sail. You have to trust your crew, and the crew needs to trust their skipper.

My parents and I arrived at American Yacht Club by 10 a.m. on that first day. I had mixed feelings seeing the Ideal 18s lined up at the dock, sails fluttering, and knowing some challenging weather was predicted for the day. The sailors and the race committee congregated under a big white tent where we received information about the events of the first day, and boats and crew members were assigned. Ironically, the boat I would skipper was named *Atlanta*, reminding me of how far I had come since my therapy at Shepherd Center in Atlanta. Cliff and an amputee would be my crew.

From the corner of the tent, a familiar voice said, "Oh my God. Is that you, Chris?" It was Grace, a girl I had sailed with at Longshore. I hadn't seen her since my accident, but it felt like old times seeing her again. With a twinkle in her eye and excitement in her voice, she commented to her own crew, "We've got our competition. Chris is back."

The tide was going out, so the ramp to the dock was steep. Volunteers wheeled the sailors, including myself, down the ramp. I was one of the only ones to have family and friends there to support me and help me get loaded onto the boat, which was quite a procedure. First, it took several people to hoist me out of my chair and sit me on the edge of the dock with my feet over the side of the boat. Then my mom got in the boat facing me. She put her arms snugly under my armpits, wrapped them around me, and pulled me into a seat installed in the boat solely for my purpose.

"That wasn't so bad," a volunteer remarked from the dock.

"For who?" my mom responded with a chuckle. She made it look easy, but it took a lot of strength. Once in the seat, my chest was strapped and buckled into the boat tightly. A gait belt was tied around my legs above the knees to secure them and keep them from flopping back and forth. Being strapped in gave me some concern. I would not be able to release the buckle myself if the boat went over, which was opposite of what I'd been taught: get out from under the boat quickly. In the event we capsized, Cliff would have to release me and then my life jacket would inflate when touched by water—a very scary thought for both of us.

Cliff didn't let on until after the third race that he was nervous about this too. Apparently, he couldn't sleep the night before wondering if this was a crazy idea. If you have ever sailed in high winds and capsized like I have, you'd understand the fear. It's hard enough to manage keeping your own self safe, let alone helping another person when a boat goes over. Next, my left hand, which is the more functioning of the two, was secured with Velcro to the tiller using "Active Hands," which I use when lifting weights. It has a mitten open on one side with a Velcro strap that goes around my wrist and over the mitten. The strap is pulled tight and curls around my hand, pulling it into a fist and allowing me to hold onto weights, or the tiller in this case.

Once the boats were rigged, all disabled sailors were secured, and the committee blew its horn, we headed out of the harbor. Here I was at the helm, five years and 310 days since having last stepped foot on a sailboat. This moment had been put off for a long, long time out of fear, anxiety, and uncertainty. But today I had hope and a determination like never before as we sailed away from the dock out into Long Island Sound. My mom's voice hollered and wavered a bit, "Good luck, Chris!" Later, she expressed how emotional it was to watch me sail off. It just seemed so normal.

While a Windward Leeward race was set up, I sailed around the starting line, checking the wind and talking with Cliff about tactics. What had earlier seemed like a lifetime ago now felt like yesterday. From an onlooker's perspective, I probably appeared normal, and I actually felt like myself, like the old Chris O'Brien. It was quickly apparent that I hadn't lost my sailing skills, but I did have to rely on my crew to help me visually. As a skipper, you need to constantly shift your body to see other boats and get into position on the starting line. I couldn't do that, which made me feel somewhat vulnerable.

Despite having good eyesight, I felt visually impaired. Due to being strapped in, I couldn't shift my body. This was a bit unnerving for me, especially on the starting line. Skippers are all figuring out which end of the line is favored, and the boats are so close to each other you could reach out and touch a crew member on another boat. There's a five-minute warning horn, then a one-minute warning, skippers are yelling "Starboard," then a countdown from ten, and finally the starting gun goes off. The start of a race is pretty stressful even for an able-bodied person. So for me, without that peripheral vision, and having to rely on my crew, the first start was a bit stressful. At the same time, it was exhilarating.

During the first race, the wind was fairly calm, and we came in tenth place. I was okay with being mid-fleet in the beginning. The second race went off without a hitch, but the wind had picked up to 15 knots. The Race Committee put up a Romeo Flag, which told the boats they were required to reef their mainsail. We didn't have a reef line, so Cliff had to jury rig one using a rope lying around in the boat.

Reefing a mainsail results in less sail space, a flatter boat, and less flogging of the sail.

The third race that first day tested my nerves. The wind howled and became very shifty. As I headed downwind and rounded the mark on a broad reach, the wind took hold of the boat. Being on the leeward side, my back went underwater, and water poured over me and into the boat. At that moment, I imagined the boat capsizing and being stuck underneath. Cliff grabbed the mainsheet and let the sail out, which leveled the boat. His face was a combination of fear and business. Cliff was not scared for himself, but for my safety. After that, I was done in for the day. As we sailed back to the dock, Cliff assured me that he would not let anything bad happen out there. We went through a few possible scenarios and discussed safety measures he would take to keep myself and the other crew member safe.

We ended the day with a 10th, 8th, and 14th. Okay, but I wanted to do better than that even if it was my first time back out on the water. After the race, we sat on the patio overlooking the harbor with beers and "Dark and Stormies" with my family and friends, talking about the races. Sailors love to rehash what went well and what didn't go well after a regatta. It felt like old times. That, coupled with the taste of saltwater on my skin and lips, brought back an indescribable nostalgia.

On day two, gusty winds had me rehashing again the first day's terrifying moment when my back hit the water. Not being able to release myself from the seat, not being in control, made me uneasy, and what a huge responsibility that was for Cliff. It didn't help that once we were out of the harbor, the Race Committee postponed the first race due to the wind gusts and shifts.

We had a new crew, a guy named Colin with muscular dystrophy. He was an experienced sailor from Vermont. Sitting in one position in an 18-foot boat for two hours waiting for the race to start was a long time for all of us. I hadn't drunk much water because I can't just stand up and pee off the boat like I used to. My rear end was getting fatigued, and I was eager to get on with the races.

Finally, the committee boat started the countdown. That day we got a 13th in the first race due to a bad start, but that got me fired up. Cliff, Colin, and I began talking tactics. At the start of the second race, I was pumped. "Let's do this, guys." And we did. With a 6th place and a 9th place, we had improved. All the while, my mom and dad, Cliff's wife, and Meg were watching me and cheering me on from a power boat. I sensed their pride and excitement for seeing me back in my old element, which made me want to do even better.

The third day started out in typical Long Island Sound fashion with no wind at all. So once again we sat around in boats, but this time waiting for the wind to blow. Our sails sat still. It can be feast or famine on Long Island Sound. Finally, after another waiting game of two hours, the first race began. I felt great, strong and ready to race. We were really talking like a team. My starts and my feel for the Ideal 18 were better, and it showed. That day, I would get a 5th and a 4th.

When I crossed the finish line in 4th place on the last race, I could hear my mom and friends hooting and hollering for me. I felt a sense of accomplishment as we sailed back into the harbor after the last race. What had seemed like an incredibly daunting task turned out to be feasible. My world opened up that weekend to other sailing events. My outlook, while always good, was more positive than ever. I could do anything I set my mind to now.

CHAPTER 28

We're Good

In three words I can sum up everything
I've learned about life: it goes on.
—ROBERT FROST[35]

s a little boy, I would look out the window of my red cape house and see a big yard, my playground. I can picture the huge lawn with its green grass, swing set, and slide where my brother and my friends would run around and play ball, where our imaginations took over for hours at a time. We were Batman and Robin, cops and robbers, cowboys and Indians, Power Rangers, Superman. I can still picture the backyard when, years later, I was a teenager. It became a place where friends congregated for touch football games, barbeques, and Thanksgiving brunch after the high school rivalry football game, and other family events.

My backyard was a safe haven and a symbol for growing up in a suburban town with few worries in the world. Today I look out the window of my house differently. I see beyond the grass, the imagination of my youth, to the events that have made me who I am today. There is a world of opportunity out there for me. In May of 2018, I will be a Harvard graduate—unimaginable prior to my accident—and go on to have a career helping others in similar situations. My rehabilitation continues at Kennedy Krieger and (through a grant) at Project Walk in New Hampshire, where the focus is on retraining the nervous system and strengthening muscles. I get physically stronger every day. I have dreams, things on my bucket list, and goals for my future.

Someday I will have a career and be independent. Maybe someday I will even have a family and kids of my own. Someday I *will* walk again. Right now, I'm not exactly sure how it will all go, but that is no different from how life has been for the past six years, and look at how far I've come. What happens over the next year, five years, ten years will be a result of technological advances for spinal cord injuries paired with my continued faith, hope, and determination to walk again. I can say with honesty and integrity that I'm good, my family is good…we're good.

My life has truly just begun.

PART VI

HELPFUL RESOURCES

Websites:
Americans with Disabilities; ADA National Network; www.ada.gov
Bureau of Rehabilitation Services www.ct.gov/brs/
Christopher and Dana Reeve Foundation www.christopherreeve.org/
Gaylord Rehabilitation www.gaylord.org
Kennedy Krieger Institute kennedykrieger.org/patient-care/
diagnoses-disorders/spinal-cord-injury-and-paralysis
Medicaid www.medicare.gov
Obie Harrington-Howes Foundation Inc. www.nepva.org/
downloads/CT%20Grant.pdf
Project Walk www.projectwalk.com/About-Us/Project-Walk-
History.asp
Quadriplegia & Body Temperature Regulation
Rhode Island Hospital www.rhodeislandhospital.org/
Shepherd Center www.shepherd.org
Supplemental Security Income Supplemental Security Income

Other information for caregivers to consider:

1. Research rehabilitation hospitals immediately after the accident.

2. Work with Social Security to get on Medicaid.

3. Fully understand the benefits you can receive from Supplemental Security Income (SSI); visit the website and find out whether you qualify.

4. Have a caseworker, follow up with SSI, and insist on getting more information.

5. When you have an injury, demand an air mattress, which will help prevent getting bed sores.

6. Don't place blame on the injured person for the accident; they did not choose this for themselves.

7. Understand medications and side effects.

8. Look into ramps to be paid for by the state; quotes are mandatory.

9. Apply for therapy grants.

10. When traveling by plane, people with power chairs need an alternate chair for entering the plane. The chairs are put with the baggage and can be damaged. With a manual chair, take the wheels off and bring them on the plane.

11. Seek home therapy after discharge; Gaylord helped set this up for Chris.

12. Shower chairs are usually not covered by insurance but are an out-of-pocket expense.

13. Get bone density tests; the injured person should be using a standing frame at the onset of injury and be on some kind of supplement D and B12.

14. Be careful in hot and cold temperatures; quadriplegics' body temperature is not 98.6 like the average person. Quads should not be out in temperatures above 90 degrees since

they do not sweat. Their body temperature will rise, which is called poikilothermic, and they can become hyperthermic. If that does happen, use a cold compress on the forehead to bring the body temp down. Quads should not go out for long periods of time in cold weather either as they can become hypothermic.[36]

15. Apply for handicap driving insurance.

16. Ease off on medications when possible; in the beginning you can't really change the meds, but talk with a neurologist about a plan to reduce medications.

17. Acupuncture therapy can promote better blood flow.

18. Acne can result from trauma—use baby wash and/or go see a dermatologist.

19. Insurance after age twenty-six can be an issue. Make sure to discuss options with insurance company.

20. Don't let driver's license expire.

ABOUT THE AUTHOR

With twenty years of teaching experience, Meg Keeshan McGovern currently teaches Middle School Language Arts. It's no surprise that her favorite genre to teach is memoir, and she loves to write with her students. While *We're Good* is her first non-fiction memoir to be published, she has other work in progress. Her children, Bill and Peter are 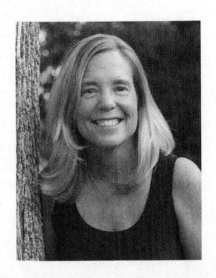 grown and live in Virginia and Vermont. She resides in Connecticut with her husband, Brian and yellow lab, Gia.

Notes

1. "Eleanor Roosevelt Quotes - BrainyQuote." https://www.brainyquote.com/authors/eleanor_roosevelt. 28 Dec. 2017.

2. "Growth That Starts from Thinking « Eleanor Roosevelt| This I Believe." 31 Jul. 2009, http://thisibelieve.org/essay/16936/. 18 Jul. 2017.

3. "Be Not Afraid Lyrics - Religious Music - LyricsBox." https://www.lyricsbox.com/religious-music-be-not-afraid-lyrics-xx3p3hq.html. 18 Jul. 2017.

4. "The Vineyard Race | Stamford Yacht Club." 2013. 20 Jul. 2015 <http://www.stamfordyc.com/node/537>

5. "Winners never quit and quitters never win. - Vince Lombardi ...." https://www.brainyquote.com/quotes/vince_lombardi_122285. 28 Dec. 2017.

6. "Quote by Ernest Hemingway: "The world breaks everyone and ...." https://www.goodreads.com/quotes/6592630-the-world-breaks-everyone-and-afterward-many-are-strong-at. 28 Dec. 2017.

7. "Without friends no one would choose to live, though he had all other ..." <http://www.quotationspage.com/quote/1485.html>

8. "God could not be everywhere, and therefore he made mothers ...." https://www.brainyquote.com/quotes/rudyard_kipling_118509. 28 Dec. 2017.

9. "Helen Keller - Brainy Quote." https://www.brainyquote.com/quotes/helen_keller_121382. 28 Dec. 2017.

10. "Using A Halo Brace After Spinal Cord Injury - Care Guide." 2007. 22 Jan. 2015 <http://www.drugs.com/cg/using-a-halo-brace-after-spinal-cord-injury.html>

11. "Quadriplegia : Quadriplegic - Apparelyzed." 2011. 27 Jan. 2015 <http://www.apparelyzed.com/quadriplegia-quadriplegic.html>

12. "Spinal Cord Injury Levels & Classification." 2003. 27 Jan. 2015 <http://www.sci-info-pages.com/levels.html>

13. "'Coughalator' brings hope to spinal cord injury patients ..." 2010. 9 Feb. 2015 <https://www.neura.edu.au/news-events/news/coughalator-brings-hope-spinal-cord-injury-patients>

14. "What is a tracheostomy? - Johns Hopkins Medicine." 2008. 9 Feb. 2015 <http://www.hopkinsmedicine.org/tracheostomy/about/what.html>

15. "Quote - The present is the ever moving shadow that divides ..." <http://quotationsbook.com/quote/32235/>

16. "Gaylord / Wallingford - Gaylord Hospital." 2013. 15 Feb. 2015 <http://www.gaylord.org/general-information/locations/gaylord-wallingford.aspx>

17. "Bladder Management - Spinal Cord Injury - Paralysis ..." 2014. 9 Mar. 2015 <http://www.christopherreeve.org/bladder>

18. "Spinal Cord Injury Bladder Management." http://www.sci-info-pages.com/bladder.html. 28 Dec. 2017.

19. "One who gains strength by overcoming obstacles ... - BrainyQuote." <http://www.brainyquote.com/quotes/quotes/a/albertschw155978.html>

20. "The most wasted of all days is one without laughter. - Goodreads." <http://www.goodreads.com/quotes/4891-the-most-wasted-of-all-days-is-one-without-laughter>

21. "Ekso Bionic Eksoskeleton - Gaylord.org." <https://www.gaylord. org/Our-Programs/Spinal-Cord/Ekso-Bionic-Eksoskeleton>

22. "Quote - Hope is the companion of power, and mother of success; for ..." <http://quotationsbook.com/quote/19499/>

23. "Kennedy Krieger Institute |." 9 Mar. 2015 <http://www. kennedykrieger.org/>

24. "We can't direct the wind, but we can adjust the... - Goodreads." http://www.goodreads.com/quotes/495000-we-can-t-direct- the-wind-but-we-can-adjust-the. 18 Jul. 2017.

25. "Quote - God grant me the serenity to accept the things I cannot ..." <http://quotationsbook.com/quote/5766/>

26. "Peace Prayer of St. Francis of Assisi :: Catholic News Agency." https://www.catholicnewsagency.com/resources/saints/saints/ peace-prayer-of-st-francis-of-assisi. 28 Dec. 2017.

27. "Anchor | Definition of Anchor by Merriam-Webster." 2005. 16 May. 2016 <http://www.merriam-webster.com/dictionary/ anchor>

28. "Compass dictionary definition | compass defined – Your Dictionary." http://www.yourdictionary.com/compass. 18 Jul. 2017.

29. "When one door closes, another opens; but we often ... - Brainy Quote." https://www.brainyquote.com/quotes/alexander_ graham_bell_409116. 28 Dec. 2017.

30. "Christopher Cross Lyrics - Sailing - A-Z Lyrics." http://www. azlyrics.com/lyrics/christophercross/sailing.html. 31 Jan. 2017.

31. "Virtual Sailing Simulator Shows Key Role of Recreation in ..." 2013. 24 Jan. 2016 <http://www.kennedykrieger.org/overview/ news/virtual-sailing-simulator-shows-key-role-recreation- spinal-cord-injury-rehabilitation>

32. "Quote - The potential of the average person is like a huge ocean ..." <http://quotationsbook.com/quote/31448/>

33. "Live as if you were to die tomorrow. Learn as if you were to live forever." <http://www.goodreads.com/quotes/2253-live-as-if-you-were-to-die-tomorrow-learn-as>

34. "A reading from the book of Sirach If you choose you can keep the ...." http://wall.st-raymond.org/wp-content/uploads/2013/01/6th-Sunday-in-Ordinary-Feb-11-and-12.pdf. 12 Feb. 2017.

35. "Thankful Quotes - BrainyQuote." https://www.brainyquote.com/quotes/topics/topic_thankful.html. 31 Jan. 2017.

36. "Quadriplegia & Body Temperature Regulation | For Caregivers." 2012. 8 Aug. 2015 <https://forcaregivers.wordpress.com/2011/07/07/body-temperature-regulation-poikilothermic-and-poikilothermia/>

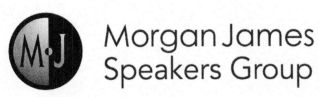

Morgan James
Speakers Group

www.TheMorganJamesSpeakersGroup.com

We connect Morgan James published authors with live and online events and audiences who will benefit from their expertise.

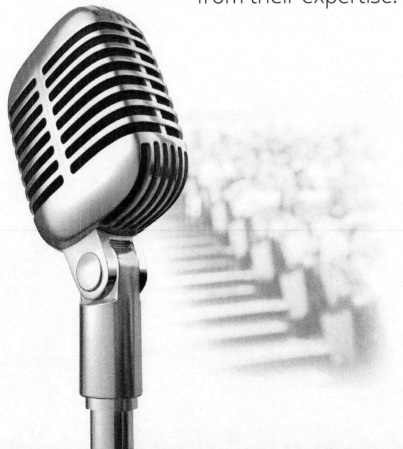

Morgan James makes all of our titles available
through the Library for All Charity Organization.

www.LibraryForAll.org